HEALTHY EATING
ON A RENAL DIET

To the memory of Peter Morris,
who pioneered home dialysis treatment and
patient education in Australia.

HEALTHY EATING ON A RENAL DIET

A Cookbook for People with Kidney Disease

Prepared by the
RENAL RESOURCE CENTRE
A Unit of Northern Sydney Area Health Service

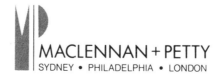

MACLENNAN + PETTY
SYDNEY • PHILADELPHIA • LONDON

First published 1991
Reprinted 1993, 1998

MacLennan & Petty Pty Limited
809–821 Botany Road, Rosebery, Sydney NSW 2018, Australia

©1991 MacLennan & Petty Pty Limited

All rights reserved including that of translation into other languages. No part of this book may be reproduced or transmitted in any form or by any means, electronic or mechanical, including photocopying, recording, or any information storage and retrieval system, without permission in writing from the publishers.

Copying for Educational Purposes

Where copies of part or the whole of this book are made under section 53B or section 53D of the Act, the law requires that records of such copying be kept and the copyright owner is entitled to claim payments.

National Library of Australia
Cataloguing-in-Publication data:

Healthy eating on a renal diet:
a cookbook for people with kidney disease.

Includes index

ISBN 0 86433 066 9

1. Kidneys—Diseases—Diet therapy—Recipes.
I. Northern Sydney Area Health Service (N.S.W.) Renal Resource Centre.

641.5631

Printed and bound in Singapore

CONTENTS

Foreword by Jo Rogers vi
Foreword by Priscilla Kincaid-Smith vii
Preface by Denise O'Shaughnessy ix
Acknowledgements x
Measures used in this book xii

1. THE COMPOSITION OF FOODS 1
2. DIET AND RECIPES FOR TREATMENT OF KIDNEY DISEASE AND PROGRESSIVE KIDNEY IMPAIRMENT 9
3. DIET AND RECIPES FOR THE PERSON ON HAEMODIALYSIS 55
4. DIET AND RECIPES FOR THE PERSON ON CONTINUOUS AMBULATORY PERITONEAL DIALYSIS (CAPD) 93
5. DIET FOR THE PERSON WITH A KIDNEY TRANSPLANT 127
6. DIET AND FOOD PREPARATION FOR CHILDREN WITH KIDNEY DISEASE 133
7. DIET FOR PERSONS WITH KIDNEY STONES .. 153

Appendices—nutrient composition of recipes
  1. Low-protein recipe analysis 157
  2. Haemodialysis recipe analysis 158
  3. CAPD recipe analysis 165
  4. Children's recipe analysis 169

Index 177

FOREWORD

If you are one of the many people with kidney disease, *Healthy Eating on a Renal Diet* will help to blow away your anxieties and negative feelings about 'being on a diet'.

Our food must be in harmony with our body. Many medical conditions, including kidney disease, affect the way our body works and this often means that we need to change our diet to maintain the diet–body harmony.

Understanding the changes in your body, and something about food and nutrition, will help you to make healthy food choices to fit in with your particular needs.

Healthy Eating on a Renal Diet provides this information in an easy-to-read form.

The different varieties of kidney disease are explained and each is accompanied by nutrition information, meal planning and cooking tips and recipes. There is a special section for children with kidney disease.

Our multicultural society is catered for with guidelines about favourite foods for many ethnic groups.

The recipes are certainly good enough to share with your family and friends and suggestions are included about the use of these foods for family meals and entertaining. There are also guidelines for those who like to eat out.

Healthy Eating on a Renal Diet has been written by dietitians and other health professionals who have worked with patients in many centres. They have been joined by home economists and food consultants to produce a book which promotes healthy and enjoyable eating for the many people with kidney disease. Good nutrition is the foundation for good health. Enjoy maintaining your diet–body harmony by using *Healthy Eating on a Renal Diet*.

Jo Rogers
National Chairperson,
Australian Nutrition Foundation.

FOREWORD

Patients with renal disease very frequently need to give careful attention to their diet and be well informed on the content of different dietary substances in foods. This excellent book provides just the sort of information that such patients need. My patients often ask me for the sort of information contained here and up until now, there really has not been anything suitable available. I am sure that this book will fill the gap very well indeed.

It can be very tedious to have to watch one's diet on a long-term basis and a ready reference in which one can look up, not only the composition of the different foods, but also a number of imaginative menus to make things a little more interesting, will lighten the load that our renal patients have to carry in organizing their daily lives.

I commend this book both to nephrologists who can make their patients aware of it and to patients with renal disease.

Priscilla Kincaid-Smith
Professor, Department of Medicine,
University of Melbourne.
Director, Department of Nephrology,
Royal Melbourne Hospital, Victoria,
Australia.

PREFACE

Cookbooks abound but producing meals that are both appetising and in keeping with dietary recommendations has presented a special challenge to those with kidney disease. In particular, this task has called upon not only culinary skills but also knowledge of dietetics and nutrition.

The successful treatment of kidney disease relies on both medical and dietary management. Adherence to the special dietary guidelines prescribed by renal physicians and dietitians is an essential ingredient in the recipe for a healthy and active life.

The idea for this book was conceived in response to the ever-present need for assistance. Patients and cooks alike wanted recipes in keeping with their lifestyles and tastes. They also wanted to understand the rationale behind their diets. With each form of treatment, a new diet followed. It was evident that a cookbook tailor-made for kidney patients was needed.

With the encouragement of the Renal Resource Centre, a small group of renal dietitians collaborated to write such a book. After many hours of work, over many months, we are delighted to present a most comprehensive guide to renal diets and an international array of recipes, each one accompanied by a nutrient composition analysis.

We trust that the book will serve readers for many years and that by understanding and following the dietary principles it outlines, they will be able to concoct their own recipes, or at least modify old favourites.

Denise O'Shaughnessy
Co-ordinator, Renal Resource Centre,
Darling Point, NSW.

ACKNOWLEDGEMENTS

The Renal Resource Centre, Darling Point, a Unit of Northern Sydney Area Health Service, wishes to thank and acknowledge the contribution and effort of the working party of dietitians who have compiled this cookbook and the support given by their Dietetics Departments and Hospitals.

Margaret Allman PhD, BSc, Dip Nutr Diet, MDAA,
Royal Prince Alfred Hospital, Camperdown, NSW.
Human Nutrition Unit, Sydney University.

Linda Cumines BSc, Dip Nutr Diet, MDAA,
Lidcombe Hospital, NSW.
St Vincent's Hospital, Darlinghurst, NSW.

Kim Kelson BSc, Dip Nutr Diet, MDAA,
Royal Newcastle Hospital, NSW.

Andrea Mortensen BSc, Dip Nutr Diet, MDAA,
Royal Alexandra Hospital for Children, Camperdown, NSW.

Helen O'Connor BSc, Dip Nutr Diet, MDAA,
Royal Prince Alfred Hospital, Camperdown, NSW.

Helen Ward BSc, Dip Nutr Diet, MDAA,
Royal North Shore Hospital, St Leonards, NSW

For coordination of the project, thanks are due to:

Denise O'Shaughnessy, B.Soc.Stud.
Co-ordinator, Renal Resource Centre,
Darling Point, NSW

Special thanks for the initiation of this project is owed to Julie Blyth B.S.W. and Patsy Trethowan R.N., Royal North Shore Hospital, St Leonards, NSW.

Thanks is also due for the contributions of:

Mandy Arnold BSc, Dip Nutr Diet, MDAA, Lismore Base Hospital, NSW.

Acknowledgements

Margaret Holiday BSc, Dip Nutr Diet, MDAA, Prince Henry Hospital, Little Bay, NSW.

Sue Ranner BSc, Dip Nutr Diet, MDAA, Prince Henry Hospital, Little Bay, NSW.

Margaret Stewart, Home Economist, Royal Prince Alfred Hospital, Camperdown, NSW.

We are indebted for recipe testing to:

The Australian Women's Weekly
The Australian Gaslight Co.
Sheila Keating of Ryde Catering College

We also wish to acknowledge the Dietitians' Association of Australia (NSW Branch) and the Australian Kidney Foundation for their assistance with funding.

For their invaluable assistance in typing the manuscript, we thank:

Therese Merriman, Tubemakers of Australia Ltd
Noelene Williams, Royal Prince Alfred Hospital.

THE MEASURES USED IN THIS BOOK

The recipes in this book give metric weights and measures. The following tables should help make your cooking as easy as possible.

TABLE OF STANDARD MEASURES

Item	Measure	Weight
Baking powder	1 teaspoon	4g
Breadcrumbs, dried	1 cup	125g
Cheese, grated	1 cup	125g
Cinnamon	2 tablespoons	10g
Cocoa	1 cup	90g
Coconut, dessicated	1 cup	80g
Coffee powder	1 cup	90g
Cornflakes	1 cup	30g
Cornflour	1 tablespoon	10g
Curry Powder	2 tablespoons	10g
Fat (or margarine)	1 cup	250g
Flour, white (plain/self raising)	1 cup	150g
Flour, wholemeal	1 cup	150g
Gelatine powder	1 tablespoon	15g
Golden syrup	1 cup	360g
Jelly crystals	1 cup	200g
Macaroni (cooked)	1 cup	150g
Milk powder, full fat	1 cup	110g
Milk powder, non fat	1 cup	80g
Oats, rolled, raw (dry)	1 cup	125g
Rice (cooked)	1 cup	150g
Sugar (white)	1 cup	200g
Tomato paste	1 cup	250g

Measures Used in This Book

METRIC CUPS

1 cup = 250mL
½ cup = 125mL
¼ cup = 62.5mL

METRIC SPOONS

1 tablespoon = 20mL
1 teaspoon = 5mL

STANDARD SERVING UTENSILS

1 soup ladle = 250mL
1 ice-cream scoop no 16 = 90g of mashed vegetables
1 ice-cream scoop no 20 = 60g of mashed vegetables

CHAPTER

1

THE COMPOSITION OF FOODS

Foods are composed of nutrients. These nutrients are known as: protein; carbohydrate; fat; vitamins and minerals; fibre; and water. Each of these nutrients has an important role in the body.

PROTEIN

Protein facilitates tissue and muscle growth and repair, the maintenance of blood proteins and the regulation of body chemistry and function.

CARBOHYDRATE AND FAT

The major function of carbohydrate and fat is to provide energy for the body.

VITAMINS AND MINERALS

Vitamins and minerals enable us to utilize the energy from the food we eat.

FIBRE

Fibre is the indigestible component of bread, cereals, fruit, vegetables and nuts. It cannot be broken down in the human gastrointestinal tract. Fibre adds bulk to the body's waste material (this prevents constipation). Some types of fibre (particularly fruit, legume and oat fibre) appear to lower the blood cholesterol levels.

WATER

Water assists in transporting nutrients and eliminating wastes. It is essential for most of the chemical processes that occur in the body.

THE FUNCTION OF THE KIDNEYS

The kidneys perform many functions in the body. Their two major roles are:

1. Excretory role—They remove waste products, particularly the nitrogen wastes (urea and creatinine) from the proteins we eat.
2. Regulatory role—They regulate and maintain a water and salt (electrolyte) balance by both removing and absorbing water and electrolytes from the blood.

Kidneys are composed of many smaller units called nephrons. The nephrons are the working units of the kidney.

If the kidneys are impaired, water and electrolyte (e.g. sodium, potassium, phosphorus) balances are disturbed and waste nitrogen products accumulate in abnormal quantities in the blood.

Diet is therefore of major importance in the treatment of kidney disease. As your kidneys become unable to cope with normal food intake, you must modify your diet.

Each person's kidney disease and the course it takes is different. Your diet plan will take into account your individual needs.

The changes you need to make in your food and fluid intake will vary during the course of your disease. Only certain sections of this book may be applicable to you at any one time. As you change your diet, please remember the changes are designed to maintain optimum health for you at this time. It may not be a good diet for your friend or for you at some later stage. Diets are individual and what is healthy for one may not be healthy for the next.

PROTEIN MODIFICATIONS

In early kidney disease, the number of functional nephrons is reduced. During these early stages the kidney as a whole will try to maintain the normal workload by making the remaining nephrons work harder. This increased work is damaging to them and will

The Composition of Foods

lead to further kidney damage until the remaining nephrons are unable to cope.

If the protein content of the diet is reduced, less nitrogen waste products are produced and hence less work has to be done by the kidneys. That is, we reduce the work for the remaining nephrons and by doing this we prolong their life. For this reason, in early kidney disease, lowering the protein intake is important.

The low-protein diet is also used in later kidney disease when the kidneys are simply unable to cope with removing protein waste products. If protein intake is unrestricted, nitrogen waste products would accumulate in the blood leading to tiredness, loss of appetite and nausea. The protein restriction at this stage is stricter than in early kidney disease.

Dialysis is commenced when the kidneys are no longer able to cope and dietary modifications can no longer compensate for the decreased kidney function.

Dialysis (haemodialysis or peritoneal dialysis) performs a similar role to the kidneys. When dialysis is commenced a strict low-protein diet is no longer needed.

As haemodialysis is performed on an intermittent basis the levels of waste products may build up between dialysis and it may be necessary to regulate your protein intake. Your doctor or dietitian will determine how much protein is needed from the level of nitrogen wastes (creatinine, urea) in your blood.

Continuous ambulatory peritoneal dialysis (CAPD) is performed on a continuous basis. As the waste products are removed continuously you do not need to restrict your protein intake. However excessive amounts of blood proteins may be removed. This loss needs to be replaced by the diet; therefore a high protein diet needs to be followed.

POTASSIUM

Potassium restriction is only necessary when potassium levels in the blood become high. This generally occurs only in advanced kidney disease when urine output is low.

A low-potassium diet is usually needed for people undergoing haemodialysis. Due to the intermittent nature of haemodialysis, potassium levels can reach high levels between dialysis treatments.

As CAPD is a continuous dialysis, potassium restriction is generally not required. However, if CAPD is ceased for some reason, the low-potassium diet should be resumed.

HEALTHY EATING ON A RENAL DIET

SALT (Sodium Chloride)

You will notice that we have omitted salt from the recipes used in this book. High salt intakes can be associated with the development of hypertension (high blood pressure). If you already have hypertension, decreasing your salt intake may help to control it. Many renal patients have to restrict their fluid intake. Eating salty foods will make you thirsty. Restricting the amoung of salt and salty foods in your diet will help you keep to your fluid restriction.

Table salt is *sodium chloride.* You should also try to limit your intake of other sodium-rich compounds such as *monosodium glutamate* and *sodium bicarbonate* (baking soda), *except* if prescribed by your doctor.

The foods listed in the box below are very rich in salt and should therefore be avoided:

Bonox	Soya sauce
Olives	Tamari
Bovril	Marmite
Onion salt	Tomato sauce
Celery salt	Monosodium glutamate (MSG)
Pickles	Mayonnaise (commercial)
Salad dressings (commercial)	Vegemite
Sea salt	Miso
Rock salt	Meat tenderizers
Garlic salt	Worcestershire sauce
Vegetable salt	Mustard paste (commercial)
Gravox	Stock cubes

Other Hints to Help Decrease your Sodium Intake

Substitute salt-reduced or salt-free foods for the regular (high-salt) versions that you are currently using. Salt-reduced products usually contain 50% to 70% less salt.

Limit your intake of corned and processed meat and fish, e.g. ham, bacon, corned beef, devon, salami and frankfurts as these are high in salt. Choose tinned fish which contains no added salt.

When using canned vegetables, choose those brands which are labelled 'no added salt'. Use salt-free or low-salt butters and margarine.

Low Salt/High Potassium

Many new salt-reduced lines are appearing on supermarket shelves. However, sometimes potassium chloride is substituted for sodium chloride and people on potassium-restricted diets should not use these products. If you are in doubt about any low-salt products, check with you dietitian or doctor.

Flavour Without Sodium

Life without salt need not mean bored taste buds. Herbs and spices make food more tasty and attractive. Try these suggestions to enhance the flavour of your cooking.

EGGS—Black pepper, chives, onion, parsley or curry.
FISH—Lemon juice, ginger, lime juice, mixed herbs, onion and tomato, parsley, white wine.
MEATS
LAMB and MUTTON—Mint, rosemary, currant jelly, paprika, mixed herbs, oregano.
BEEF—Bay leaf, sage, homemade mustard. Add red wine to beef casseroles.
VEAL—Lemon juice, oregano, rosemary.
PORK—Garlic, coriander, apple sauce, apricot puree.
CHICKEN AND POULTRY—Mushrooms, garlic, white wine, tarragon.
STEWS AND CASSEROLES—Curry, oregano leaves, bay leaves, onion, garlic, allspice, cloves.
VEGETABLES
ASPARAGUS—Lemon juice.
BRUSSEL SPROUTS AND CABBAGE—Oil, vinegar plus a pinch of dry mustard, black pepper.
CARROTS—Honey, cinnamon, parsley.
CAULIFLOWER—Nutmeg.
GREEN BEANS—Marjoram, lemon juice with grated onion.
LETTUCE—Unsalted French dressing.
MARROW—Mace, ginger.
PEAS—Mint, sugar.
PUMPKIN—Nutmeg, black pepper.
POTATO—Mint, chives, parsley, onion, paprika.
TOMATO—Basil, oregano, parsley.

Special Note

Some of you may have a type of renal failure (salt-losing nephropathy) which actually increases the amount of salt you need. If you are in doubt about increasing your salt intake, check with your doctor.

THE MODIFIED FAT DIET

High blood fats (cholesterol and triglycerides) have been associated with diets high in saturated fats and cholesterol. If you have a persistently high blood cholesterol level, the result may be fatty deposits on artery walls (atherosclerosis). This leads to a reduction in the blood flow through the arteries and hence to the organs. Decreased blood to the organs damages the tissues and contributes to coronary heart disease, stroke and peripheral vascular disease.

A high intake of saturated fats, which are found predominantly in foods of animal origin, eg. butter, full cream milk and dairy foods, the fat on meat, are associated with high blood cholesterol levels.

A high intake of cholesterol, found in egg yolks, offal (except tripe), prawns and squid is also associated with elevated blood cholesterol levels.

Polyunsaturated fats (oils) found predominantly in foods of plant and fish origin do not contribute to a raised blood cholesterol level. Monounsaturated fats found in some nuts, avocados, olives and lean meats do not contribute to a raised blood cholesterol level.

In order to help maintain a normal blood cholesterol level you should:

1. Achieve and maintain an ideal body weight.
2. Reduce your saturated fat intake. Avoid butter, lard, shortening, copha and dripping. Use lean meats and remove the skin from poultry. Use low-fat dairy products and avoid cream. Reduce your intake of high-fat commercial products, e.g. pastries, chips, pies and chocolates.
3. Reduce your cholesterol intake: Restrict egg yolks to two per week. Reduce your intake of prawns and squid. Reduce your intake of offal.
4. Replace saturated fats with polyunsaturated or monounsaturated fats (if your weight is normal, remember all fats are energy dense). Use polyunsaturated margarines and cooking oils or olive and peanut oils.

The Composition of Foods

The recipes in this book incorporate polyunsaturated and monounsaturated fats in place of saturated fats. Similar modifications may be made to your own recipes. If your triglyceride level is also high, it will be necessary to limit your intake of sugars and alcohol.

CHAPTER

2

DIET AND RECIPES FOR TREATMENT OF KIDNEY DISEASE AND PROGRESSIVE KIDNEY IMPAIRMENT

The low-protein diet	10
Food preparation and cooking	12
Low-phosphorous diets	13
Eating out	14
Low-protein recipes	
Soups	17
Vegetable meals	20
Meatless meals with alternative protein	25
Main meals	28
Sauces and dressings	36
Salads	40
Desserts	43
Bread, biscuits and cakes	51

THE LOW-PROTEIN DIET

The Structure of Proteins

Proteins are made up of smaller structural units called amino acids. There are 22 amino acids in nature. Nine of these are classified as indispensible or essential. These indispensible (essential) amino acids cannot be made by the human body and hence must be supplied in the diet. The other amino acids, which can be produced by the body, are dispensible (non-essential) amino acids.

Proteins vary in both the type and quantity of amino acids. Foods that contain all the indispensible amino acids are called high biological value or complete proteins. Food with a low proportion of indispensible amino acids are called low biological value or incomplete proteins.

If a diet is low in protein it is necessary to ensure that the protein in the diet is of high biological value in order to satisfy the indispensible amino acid requirement.

COMPLETE PROTEINS
Eggs
Milk, yoghurt, cheese
Fish and seafoods
Poultry
Veal, beef, lamb and pork
These foods are high in protein and therefore quantities specified in the diet must be followed carefully.
INCOMPLETE PROTEINS
Legumes (e.g. lentils, broad beans, kidney beans, chick peas, haricot beans, soya beans, baked beans)
Nuts
Chocolate
These proteins are not used efficiently by the body and result in protein wasteage and hence high levels of protein breakdown products.

Proteins, carbohydrates and fats all contain carbon, hydrogen and oxygen. However, protein also contains nitrogen. It is this nitrogen component that needs to be removed by the kidneys. If kidney function is impaired, a high protein intake is undesirable as it increases the work load of the kidneys. A high protein intake in a person with impaired kidney function has two adverse effects: it is damaging to the existing kidney function; and it creates a build-up of the waste products of protein (urea and creatinine) in the blood. This can lead to nausea and loss of appetite.

The aim of the low-protein diet is to supply only enough protein for the body to use without providing excess. This is achieved by:

1. Reducing your total protein intake according to your body weight.
2. Ensuring that the majority of your protein comes from high biological value foods, i.e. proteins that can be utilized completely by the body with little wasteage.
3. Ensuring that your daily protein intake is evenly distributed during the day to maximize the use of the protein. The body is unable to utilize protein efficiently if it receives large amounts at once.

Energy (Kilojoules/Calories)

In order to judge if you are receiving adequate energy from your low-protein diet, watch your weight. If you are losing weight it will be necessary to increase your energy intake from foods that contain little or no protein, such as sugar and fats. The waste products of sugar and fats do not have to be removed from the body by the kidneys.

Sugars	
Sugar	Honey
Glucose	Icing
Jam	Marmalade
Syrups	Soft drinks

If you don't like sweet food, coldness and acidity (lemon juice and citric acid) will decrease the taste of sweetness in food.

Protein-Free Lollies	
Barley Sugar	Life Savers
Jelly Babies	Jelly Beans
Fruit Bonbons	Mint Leaves
Musk sticks	Jubes
Peppermints	Boiled Lollies

> **Fats and Oils**
>
> *Polyunsaturated and monounsaturated fats*
>
> Polyunsaturated margarine
> Polyunsaturated oils (e.g. sunflower, safflower)
> Olive oil
> Peanut oil
> Polyunsaturated salad oils
>
> *Saturated fats*
>
> | | |
> |---|---|
> | Butter | Copha |
> | Lard | Salad Oils |
> | Shortening | |

Remember your blood cholesterol level and try to use polyunsaturated or monounsaturated fat in preference to saturated fats.

Food Preparation and Cooking

Preparing and cooking a low-protein diet is not difficult, but requires a little care to ensure that only the correct amount of protein allowed in the diet is consumed.

There should be no trouble in fitting in with family meals as the diet will mainly affect the serving size of normal foods.

Each serve in the recipes in this chapter is equal to 30g protein. When cooking for family members who are not restricted to a low-protein diet you may need to calculate more than 1 serve per person.

The following points may help you to stick to your low-protein diet.

1. Check quantities and measure carefully all ingredients in recipes, particularly the high-protein foods (meat, fish, poultry, eggs, milk, cheese).
2. Take into consideration foods which contain smaller but still significant amounts of protein (bread, flour, potato, rice, pasta, corn).
3. Try to avoid the low biological value protein foods such as legumes and nuts.
4. Arrowroot and cornflour have a lower protein content than wheat flour and hence may be used in place of wheat flour, e.g.

Kidney Disease and Progressive Kidney Impairment

as thickening agents, in cakes and biscuits, coating foods prior to frying.

5. Sago and tapioca are virtually free from protein and may be served as an extra food during the day, e.g. boiled, sweetened, flavoured, added to rice dishes to give a greater quantity.
6. Cream and water mixtures act as a low-protein substitute for milk.
7. Read labels on convenience foods. Some products have increased protein levels, e.g. added milk solids, milk powder, gluten.
8. Avoid unlabelled, commercially prepared foods as the protein (and sodium) levels can be both high and variable.

LOW-PHOSPHOROUS DIETS

A low-phosphorous diet is often prescribed in addition to a low-protein diet for people with declining renal function. As foods that are high in protein are also high in phosphorous, the low-phosphorous diet is consistent with a low-protein diet and also aims to reduce the quantity of waste products that need to be filtered from the blood by the kidneys.

The main sources of phosphorous in the diet are milk and other dairy products including cheese, yoghurt and ice cream. The quantity of these foods in the low-protein, low-phosphorous diet is limited as is the quantity of meat, fish, chicken, eggs and seafood allowed. Breads and cereals are lower in protein and phosphorous than dairy products or meat but still contain sufficient protein to require restriction of the quantity allowed. Most fruits and vegetables are very low in phosphorous and are usually allowed in unlimited quantities. Fats, oils and sugars are free of protein and phosphorous.

Many processed and convenience foods have phosphorous added to them during manufacture and must be avoided. The foods that are very high in phosphorous and must be avoided are listed below.

High-phosphorous foods

1. Brains, liver, liverwurst, rabbit, sardines, anchovies, sour cream.

2. Fish and meat pastes, and various extracts (Anchovette, Bonox, Marmite, Promite), stock cubes, packet and canned soups.
3. Broad beans, lima beans, baked beans, and other dried beans.
4. Nuts, coconut, crisps, wheat germ, dried fruits and tamarinds.
5. Cola soft drinks, beer and stout.
6. Cocoa, Milo, Actavite, Ovaltine, and chocolate.

EATING OUT

Eating out on a low-protein diet requires forethought and sensible food selection. You can avoid large serves of the high-protein foods while out; or reduce your protein intake at the preceding meals. However, try not to make a habit of this as your protein intake should be distributed evenly throughout the day.

If you eat out only on a rare occasion, you can afford to be more indulgent in your choices. Discuss this with your doctor or dietitian as your current kidney function will determine the severity of the protein restriction.

If you eat out on a regular basis, you should be more rigid with your food choices.

Take-away Foods

Sensible choices are

Sandwiches or rolls
Hamburgers (avoid ones with more than one protein filling, e.g. with egg, bacon or cheese).
Small portions of chicken
Hot dogs
Fruit and fruit salads
Ice blocks
Boiled sweets

Restaurants

When having a meal at a restaurant, do not have three courses which feature protein as their main ingredient. Most people find it is easier to have:

a low-protein entree

Vegetable soup
Fruit cocktail
Melon
Avocado vinaigrette

Chinese vegetables
Vegetable vol-au-vents
Side salad

followed by

A main meal featuring protein, e.g. a small serve of meat, poultry or fish. Avoid dishes with more than one protein food such as veal cordon bleu (veal with cheese and ham)

a low-protein dessert

Fresh/stewed fruit
Fruit salad/compote and
    cream
Baked apple

Sorbet/fruit ice
Fruit fritters
Fruit crumbles and cream

FREE VEGETABLES

The vegetables listed below are on the 'free list'.

Artichokes—fresh or canned
Asparagus—fresh or canned
Beans—French—runner—
    fresh, canned or frozen
Beetroot—fresh or canned
Broccoli—fresh or frozen
Brussel sprouts—fresh or
    frozen
Cabbage—white, green or
    red
Capsicum—green, red—fresh
    or canned
Carrots—fresh, canned or
    frozen
Cauliflower—fresh or frozen
Celery

Choko
Corn—fresh, frozen, canned,
    kernels or sweet corn
Cucumber
Eggplant
Kale
Kohlrabi
Leeks
Lettuce
Marrow
Mushrooms—fresh or canned
Onions
Parsley
Parsnips
Peas, green—as allowed on
    diet

HEALTHY EATING ON A RENAL DIET

Potatoes—fresh, dehydrated or frozen	Squash
	Swede
Pumpkin	Sweet potato
Radishes	Turnip
Silver Beet	Watercress
Spinach	Zucchini

Soups

Do not forget to count the meat, barley, noodles, etc. in your homemade soup. Here are some recipes containing ingredients from the free list only.

Basic Vegetable Stock

Any mixture of chopped vegetables from the free list (pages 15–16). Add fresh ground pepper and bouquet garni (bay leaf, thyme, parsley and celery stalk wrapped in muslin). Place in cold water, bring to the boil and simmer until cooked. Strain.

Variations

Sieve or blend and thicken with cornflour. Add a bone (no meat or marrow) to give extra flavour.

Cream of Carrot Soup

SERVES 4

240g (1 cup) carrots
120g (1 medium) onion
1 tablespoon polyunsaturated oil
800mL basic vegetable stock (see above)
Pepper to taste
1 teaspoon orange rind
100mL cream
Chopped dill to garnish

Peel and dice carrots. Chop onion finely and saute with carrots in oil. Add stock and simmer until carrots are tender. Drain and reserve liquid. Blend or puree carrot and onion until smooth, then add to the liquid and reheat. Season with pepper and orange rind. Stir in cream just before serving and garnish with chopped dill.

Creamed Asparagus Soup

SERVES 4

500g (no added salt) canned asparagus
  or 1 bunch fresh asparagus (8 to 10 spears)
40g (2 level tablespoons) polyunsaturated margarine
2 teaspoons cornflour
125mL ½ cream
Pepper, lemon juice, thyme and caraway seeds to taste
Extra cream and chopped parsley for garnish

If using fresh asparagus, slice wood tip off asparagus and wash well. Place spears in a stainless steel or enamel saucepan. Just cover with cold water, bring to the boil and simmer for 3 to 4 minutes. Remove from heat and allow to stand in the water in which they were cooked for 6 to 8 minutes.

Drain the asparagus (fresh or canned) and reserve liquid. Chop asparagus spears. Melt margarine and stir in cornflour. Combine asparagus liquid, cream and enough water to make 500mL. Gradually add this to the margarine mixture, stirring over low heat. Bring to the boil, add asparagus, pepper, lemon juice, thyme and caraway seeds to taste. Simmer for 5 minutes.

Garnish with a swirl of extra cream and a sprinkle of chopped parsley.

Onion Soup

SERVES 4

480g (4 medium) onions
2 tablespoons polyunsaturated oil
800mL basic vegetable stock (see page 17)
Pepper to taste
100mL cream

Peel and slice onions thinly. Heat oil and cook onions until transparent. Add stock and pepper. Simmer for 20 minutes. Stir in cream just before serving.

Gazpacho

SERVES 4

300mL tomato juice (no added salt)
265g (2 medium) cooked tomatoes
  or 150g canned tomatoes (no added salt)
½ clove garlic, crushed
½ teaspoon chilli sauce
⅓ bunch parsley, chopped
¼ bunch fresh basil
2 teaspoons polyunsaturated oil
1 tablespoon cornflour
Freshly ground black pepper
80mL sour cream and extra basil to garnish (optional)

Mix all ingredients (except garnish) in blender and process until well combined. Serve with a swirl of sour cream and a garnish of basil if desired.

Vegetable Meals

If you are on a very low protein diet (less than 30g/day) you may use these recipes as a main meal. If you are on a higher protein intake substitute 1 serve of these dishes for 2 servings of vegetables.

Ratatouille

SERVES 2

100g (1 small) egg plant
2 tablespoons polyunsaturated oil
120g (1 medium) onion, sliced
60g (1 medium) zucchini
270g (2 medium) tomatoes
80g (1 medium) capsicum
Pinch mixed herbs
1 clove garlic, crushed

Cut eggplant into 2cm cubes, soak in cold water for 1 hour and drain. Heat oil and fry sliced onion until softened. Add eggplant, remaining chopped vegetables, herbs and garlic. Fry, stirring frequently, till cooked. Serve hot or cold.

Fried Rice

SERVES 4

60g (¼ cup) uncooked rice
120g (1 medium) onion, chopped
2 tablespoons polyunsaturated oil
60g (1 small) carrot, grated
135g (1 medium) tomato, diced
Pepper to taste
2 tablespoons shallots, chopped

Cook rice in boiling unsalted water until tender. Drain and rinse in cold water. Refrigerate for several hours. Fry onion in polyunsaturated oil until transparent, add carrot and cook until golden brown. Add tomato and cold cooked rice. Heat well and season with pepper to taste. Sprinkle with shallots just before serving.

Rice Riojana

SERVES 8

240g (1 cup) uncooked long-grain rice
40mL (2 tablespoons) polyunsaturated oil
1 clove garlic, crushed
½ teaspoon tumeric
6 shallots, chopped and separated white from green
80g (1 medium) red capsicum, chopped
250g corn kernels (no added salt)
Pepper to taste

Cook rice in boiling, unsalted water. Drain, rinse in cold water and refrigerate for several hours.

Heat oil, garlic, tumeric, white of shallot and capsicum. Cook for 3 minutes. Add corn and rice, toss well with a fork, and cook until heated. Add pepper to taste. Serve sprinkled with the green part of the shallots.

Vegetable Cakes

SERVES 4

40mL (2 tablespoons) polyunsaturated oil
120g (1 medium) onion, diced
200g (1 cup) mixed vegetables, boiled
40mL (2 tablespoons) cream
Cornflour for rolling
Extra polyunsaturated oil

Heat the oil and saute the onion until tender. Mash vegetables and onion together with a fork, using cream to moisten. Shape into 8 patties and toss in cornflour. Fry until golden brown in hot oil.

Stuffed Capsicum

SERVES 2

80g (1 medium) capsicum
60g (½ medium) onion, chopped
1 clove garlic, crushed
Pinch paprika
20g (1 tablespoon) polyunsaturated margarine
60g (¼ cup) uncooked rice
125mL (½ cup) basic vegetable stock (page 17)
30g pineapple pieces, drained well
Extra margarine, melted

Halve the capsicum, remove seeds and membrane, and steam until tender. Gently fry onion, garlic and paprika in margarine. Add rice, stock and pineapple. Cover and cook for 20 to 25 minutes. Fill capsicum halves with rice mixture, brush with melted margarine and bake in a moderate oven (180°C) for 15 minutes.

Vegetable Pie

SERVES 6

540g (4 medium) tomatoes
160g (4 sticks) celery
120g (2 small) carrots
480 (4 medium) onions
120g (1 cup) green beans
375mL (1½ cups) basic vegetable stock (page 17)
Mixed herbs
½ teaspoon ground marjoram
10g (1 tablespoon) cornflour
280g (1½ cups) mashed potato
20g (1 tablespoon) polyunsaturated margarine
Parlsey to garnish

Coarsely chop the vegetables, place in a saucepan and cover with stock. Add the herbs and marjoram, bring to the boil and simmer for 3 to 5 minutes or until tender. Thicken with cornflour mixed with a little water. Pour into a heatproof dish and top with mashed potato. Brush with melted margarine and bake in a moderate oven (180°C) until golden brown, approximately 30 minutes. Garnish with parsley.

Variation

Substitute 2 teaspoons curry powder for herbs.

Vegetable Croquettes

SERVES 8

20mL (1 tablespoon) polyunsaturated oil
120g (1 medium) onion, finely diced
1 tablespoon curry powder
40g (1 stick) celery, finely diced
270g (3 medium) potatoes, boiled and mashed
240g (1 cup) pumpkin, boiled and mashed
40g (2 tablespoons) polyunsaturated margarine
100g 91 cup) dry breadcrumbs
Polyunsaturated oil for deep frying

Heat the oil and saute the onion until tender. Add curry powder, celery and cook for approximately 1 minute. Remove from heat. Mash the potato and pumpkin together with margarine. Add to the onion mixture and combine well. Shape into 8 patties and coat in breadcrumbs. Refrigerate for a few hours. Deep fry in hot oil until golden brown.

Noodle–Vegetable Medley

SERVES 4

20g (½ cup) noodles or macaroni
¼ cup each of chopped onion, celery, capsicum,
    carrots and green beans
60mL (3 tablespoons) polyunsaturated oil
135g (1 medium) tomato, peeled and chopped
Pinch basil and oregano

Cook pasta in boiling, unsalted water. Fry chopped vegetables in hot oil for 4 minutes. Add tomato and herbs. Simmer 5 minutes. Toss in cooked noodles or macaroni and heat through.

Vegetable Curry

SERVES 8

200g mixed dried fruit
20mL (1 tablespoon) polyunsaturated oil
240g (2 medium) onions, diced
3 cloves garlic, crushed
2 tablespoons curry powder
Pinch chilli powder
½ teaspoon garam marsala
180g (2 medium) potatoes, chopped
200g (2 large) carrots, chopped
120g (1 cup) green beans
120g (½ cup) pumpkin, chopped (optional)
750mL (3 cups) no added salt tomato juice

Soak dried fruit in cold water for 30 minutes. Heat oil and fry onion and garlic until transparent. Add curry, chilli and garam marsala. Cook for 1 minute. Add vegetables and tomato juice. Simmer for 30 minutes. Drain fruit and add to curry. Cook, uncovered, until thickened.

Savoury Stuffed Tomatoes

SERVES 4

540g (4 medium) tomatoes
40g (2 tablespoons) polyunsaturated margarine, for frying
60g (½ medium) onion, chopped
40g (4 tablespoons) breadcrumbs
20mL (1 tablespoon) lemon juice
Pinch sage
Pepper to taste

Cut tops off tomatoes and scoop out pulp. Roughly chop pulp. Heat margarine and fry onion until soft. Combine with the chopped pulp, breadcrumbs, lemon juice, pepper and sage. Fill tomato shells with this mixture. Bake in a moderate oven (180°C) until cooked— approximately 15 minutes.

Meatless Meals with Alternative Protein

All the main meals in the following section contain protein. Use these as a '30g' meat serve.

Macaroni cheese

SERVES 6

120g (1½ cups) uncooked macaroni
1 quantity of white sauce (see below)
135g (1 medium) tomato, chopped
120g grated cheese
Paprika
½ cup shallots, chopped

White sauce

30g polyunsaturated margarine
3 tablespoons cornflour
Pepper
600mL (2¼ cups) water
200mL (¾ cup) cream

Cook macaroni in boiling, unsalted water. Meanwhile, make the white sauce (see below). Combine cooked macaroni, white sauce and tomato. Place in ovenproof dish, sprinkle with cheese and paprika. Bake in a moderate oven (180°C) for 15 minutes. Garnish with chopped shallots.

White sauce
Melt margarine, add cornflour and pepper and cook, stiring constantly, until well blended. Mix cream and water. Stir a little of this liquid into the cornflour mixture to form a smooth paste. Add remaining liquid and cook until thickened.

Potato and Carrot Pancakes

SERVES 4

500g (5 to 6 medium) potatoes, peeled
240g (4 small) carrots, peeled
30g (¼ cup) self-raising flour
Pinch of baking powder
Pinch of pepper
2 60g eggs, beaten
polyunsaturated margarine for greasing

Cut potatoes and carrots into pieces and boil for 20 minutes, or until tender. Drain and mash. Add flour, baking powder, pepper and eggs. Grease pan with margarine and place over medium heat. Place one tablespoon of mixture into the pan, flatten with an egg slice, and fry until brown underneath (approximately 2 minutes) then turn and cook other side. Repeat with the remaining mixture.

Spanish Omelette

Serves 4

1 tablespoon polyunsaturated margarine
100g (1 small) chopped onion
50g (1 small) chopped capsicum
4 × 60g eggs
¼ teaspoon paprika
½ teaspoon pepper
1 tablespoon chopped shallots
Chilli to taste
100mL (⅓ cup) water
100g (1 small) chopped tomato

Melt margarine in a frying pan. Fry onion and capsicum until tender. Mix eggs, paprika, pepper, shallots, chilli and water. Add this mixture to the pan. Place tomato on top of omelette mixture. When nearly set, fold omelette over and maintain on a moderate heat until cooked.

Kidney Disease and Progressive Kidney Impairment

Parsley Scrambled Eggs

SERVES 6

5 × 60g eggs
Pinch pepper
80mL (⅓ cup) cream
1 tablespoon polyunsaturated margarine
1 teaspoon chopped parsley

Beat eggs lightly. Add pepper and cream and mix well. Melt margarine in a saucepan. Add egg mixture and cook, stirring occasionally. Garnish with parsley.

Main Meals

Veal Marengo

SERVES 4

150g veal steak
80g (1 small) tomato, sliced
2 teaspoons parsley, chopped
30g mushrooms, sliced
80g (1 small) onion, sliced
250mL (1 cup) basic vegetable stock (see page 17)
½ teaspoon thyme

Chop veal into 2.5cm cubes. Place all ingredients into a small casserole dish and barely cover with vegetable stock. Cover and cook in a moderate oven (180°C) until meat is tender (approximately 45 minutes).

Beef Curry

SERVES 4

150g beef steak
120g (1 medium) onion, chopped
20g (1 tablespoon) polyunsaturated margarine
2 teaspoons curry powder
200mL (¾ cup) pineapple juice
½ apple
1 tablespoon capsicum, finely diced
2 teaspoons cornflour

Cut beef into 2.5 cm cubes. Saute chopped onion in margarine over medium heat. Add curry powder and beef. When beef is browned, add pineapple juice. When heated through, add chopped apple and capsicum and simmer for 1 hour. Mix cornflour with a little water and stir into beef. Heat till curry thickens.

Braised Steak

SERVES 4

150g stewing steak
Cornflour
20mL (1 tablespoon) polyunsaturated oil
120g (1 medium) onion
Pinch pepper
2 bay leaves
½ teaspoon chopped parsley
125mL (½ cup) basic vegetable stock (see page 17)

Cut meat into 2.5cm cubes and coat in cornflour. Fry in oil until browned. Place in an ovenproof dish with sliced onion, pepper, bay leaves, parsley and stock. Cover and bake in a moderate oven (180°C) for 1 hour or until meat is tender.

Savoury Meatballs

SERVES 4

160g finely minced beef
80g (1 small) onion, chopped
1 teaspoon parsley, chopped
40mL (2 tablespoons) fresh tomato puree
¼ teaspoon pepper
40mL (2 tablespoons) polyunsaturated oil
2 cups canned, peeled salt-free tomatoes
1 clove garlic, crushed
½ teaspoon oregano
190mL (¾ cup) water
1 tablespoon cornflour (optional)

Mix minced beef, onion, parsley, tomato puree and pepper. Mould into 20 balls and gently brown in hot oil. Remove meatballs, pour off excess oil from pan. Add tomatoes, garlic and oregano (do not drain tomatoes). Break up tomatoes with a spoon. Simmer for five minutes. Add water and meatballs. Cover and simmer 20 minutes or until meatballs are cooked. Thicken sauce with cornflour mixed with a little water if desired.

Cabbage Rolls

SERVES 4

4 large cabbage leaves

Filling

2 tablespoons cornflour
⅓ cup mixed vegetables, boiled
20mL (1 tablespoon) tomato sauce
20mL (1 tablespoon) water
125g minced meat

Sauce

350mL (1⅓ cups) water
1 tablespoon grated lemon rind
40mL (2 tablespoons) tomato paste
1 pinch mixed herbs

Steam or boil cabbage leaves until soft (about 3 minutes). Cut hard core from base of the leaves. Combine all the filling ingredients and place ¼ of the filling on the core end of each leaf. Roll up each leaf, tucking in edges to seal the package. Place in an ovenproof dish.

Sauce

Combine sauce ingredients and pour over the rolls (sauce can be thickened with 1 to 2 teaspoons of cornflour mixed with 1 tablespoon of water if desired). Bake in a moderate oven (180°C) for 25 to 30 minutes.

Meat Loaf

SERVES 4

Polyunsaturated margarine
160g finely minced beef
60g (½ medium) onion, chopped
1 teaspoon parsley, chopped
2 tablespoons fresh tomato puree
¼ teaspoon pepper
2 teaspoons mixed herbs

Grease an 8 × 26cm bar pan with margarine. Mix all ingredients and press into greased bar pan. Bake in a moderate oven (180°C) for 45 minutes or until well browned.

Bolognese Sauce

SERVES 6

200g minced meat
200mL (¾ cup) fresh tomato puree
20mL (1 tablespoon) polyunsaturated oil
40g (½ small) onion, finely chopped
20g (¼ medium) capsicum, finely chopped
¼ teaspoon pepper
¼ teaspoon mixed herbs
½ teaspoon sugar
¼ teaspoon paprika

Combine all the ingredients in a saucepan. Bring to the boil and simmer gently for 1 to 1½ hours. Serve with 1 cup cooked pasta per person.

Lamb Shish Kebabs

SERVES 4

100g lamb
320g (4 small) onions
400g (4 small) tomatoes
80g (1 medium) green capsicum
80g (1 medium) red capsicum
4 rings fresh or canned pineapple

Cut the lamb into 2.5cm cubes. Quarter the onions and tomatoes. Cut the capsicum and pineapple into 2.5cm squares. Alternate the different ingredients on 8 skewers. The kebabs may be barbequed or grilled until the meat is cooked.

Chicken Slice

SERVES 8

Base

> 60g (¾ cup) uncooked macaroni
> 2 tablespoons parsley, chopped
> 1 × 60g egg, lightly beaten

Filling

> 1 tablespoon cornflour
> 250mL (1 cup) basic vegetable stock
> 125g cooked chicken, sliced
> 120g (1 medium) onion, grated
> ½ cup chopped celery
> ½ teaspoon mustard powder
> ½ teaspoon thyme
> 1 tablespoon grated parmesan cheese

Base

Cook macaroni in boiling, unsalted water until tender. Drain and combine with parsley and beaten egg. Spoon evenly over the base of a pie dish.

Filling

Mix cornflour to a paste with a little stock, then add remaining stock. Add other ingredients except cheese. Pour over base and sprinkle on cheese. Bake in a moderate oven (180°C) for 15 to 20 minutes until golden brown.

Scallop Kebabs

SERVES 4

Marinade

> 1 clove garlic, crushed
> 60mL (3 tablespoons) olive oil
> 60mL (3 tablespoons) fresh lemon juice
> 30mL (1½ tablespoons) dry sherry
> 1 teaspoon marjoram
> 1 teaspoon pepper

Kebabs
>4 slices fresh pineapple
>1 green capsicum
>1 red capsicum
>16 small scallops
>8 button mushrooms
>8 cocktail onions
>Lemon wedges to garnish

Combine all marinade ingredients. Cut pineapple and capsicum into squares. Thread scallops (2 scallops per skewer), mushrooms, onion, pineapple, and capsicum on 8 bamboo skewers. Lay in a shallow dish and cover with marinade. Leave at least 30 minutes. Cook on a barbeque or under the grill, turning and basting frequently (approximately 12 minutes). Garnish with lemon wedges to serve.

Deep-fried Salmon Balls

SERVES 8

>360g (4 medium) potatoes
>120g (1 medium) sweet potato
>100g (2 small) zucchini
>30g (1 medium) celery stick
>80g (1 medium) carrot
>1 tablespoon chopped onion
>1 clove garlic, crushed
>220g (1 medium can), no added salt, salmon
>4 tablespoons parsley, chopped
>1 teaspoon mustard powder
>Juice of 1 lemon
>Pepper to taste
>Sesame seeds
>Polyunsaturated oil for deep frying

Peel and dice potatoes and sweet potato, boil until tender, then mash. Finely dice the zucchini, celery and carrot. Stir-fry, together with the onion and garlic until tender. Combine the mashed potato, salmon, parsley, mustard, lemon juice and pepper. Add the stir-fried vegetables and mix gently. Form into 32 balls, roll in sesame seeds. Heat oil (approximately 20 minutes before frying) and deep-fry until golden brown. Makes 32 balls, 4 per serve.

Chicken à la King

SERVES 6

60g (3 tablespoons) polyunsaturated margarine
80g (1 medium) green capsicum, chopped
30g mushroom, sliced
2 tablespoons cornflour
250mL (1 cup) basic vegetable stock (page 17)
120g chopped cooked chicken
250mL (1 cup) cream
Pepper

In a medium-sized saucepan melt the margarine over moderate heat. When the foam subsides add the capsicum and, stirring occasionally, cook gently until soft. Add the mushrooms and cook gently. Blend the cornflour with a little of the stock and stir in, then add the remainder of stock and chicken and cook for a few minutes. Stir in cream and pepper. Heat through but do not boil.

Curried Chicken

SERVES 6

120g (1 medium) onion, chopped
20g (¼ medium) capsicum, diced
20g (1 tablespoon) polyunsaturated margarine
1 tablespoon curry powder
135g (1 medium) tomato, chopped
1 tablespoon grated lemon rind
125mL (½ cup) water
150g cooked chicken, sliced

Fry onion and capsicum in margarine until tender. Stir in curry powder and fry for 1 minute. Add chopped tomato, lemon rind and water to pan and simmer for 10 minutes. Add sliced chicked to pan, heat through and simmer for a further 5 minutes.

Tuna Macaroni

SERVES 8

120g (1½ cup) uncooked macaroni
120g (1 medium) onion
160g (2 medium) carrots
120g (2 small) zucchini
80g (1 medium) capsicum
2 tablespoons olive oil
2½ tablespoons cornflour
250mL (1 cup) water
110g (1 small can) no added salt tuna
Juice of 1 lemon
1 tablespoon Worcestershire sauce
½ cup parsley, chopped
Pepper to taste
250mL (1 cup) cream
¼ cup puffed rice, crushed

Boil macaroni in unsalted water until tender. Drain, refresh in cool water and set aside.

While macaroni is boiling, chop onion and finely dice carrots, zucchini and capsicum. Saute in 1 tablespoon olive oil until the onions are tender. Set aside.

Mix cornflour with a little water to form a smooth paste, then add remaining water. Place over heat, stir until mixture boils and thickens. Remove from heat, add drained tuna, lemon juice, sauted vegetables, Worcestershire sauce, parsley and pepper. Mix well. Return to heat and warm, but do not boil. Stir through cream. Reheat macaroni in a pan using the remaining olive oil. Place in a serving dish and spoon tuna mixture on top of macaroni. Sprinkle with crushed puffed rice and brown for 1 minute under the griller.

Savoury Sauces and Dressings

These sauces and dressings contain small amounts of protein but up to 2 tablespoons per day can be used as an extra in your diet.

Tomato Sauce

40mL (2 tablespoons) polyunsaturated oil
240g (2 medium) onions, sliced
2 cloves garlic, crushed
600g (4 large) tomatoes
Pepper to taste
Pinch oregano
Pinch basil

Heat oil, add onion and garlic. Cook over low heat until onion softens but does not brown. Add other ingredients, cover saucepan and cook gently for 20 to 30 minutes. (Serve with spaghetti, noodles or meatballs.)

Curry Sauce

120g (1 medium) onion, chopped
40mL (2 tablespoons) polyunsaturated oil
2 teaspoons curry powder
1 tablespoon cornflour
Pepper to taste
300mL (1¼ cups) water

Fry onion in oil until brown. Add curry powder, cornflour, pepper and water. Bring to the boil, stirring constantly. Simmer gently for 10 minutes.

Sweet and Sour Sauce

90g (2 slices) canned pineapple, diced
20g (1⅓ small) carrot, sliced
40g (½ medium) capsicum, chopped
2 tablespoons salt-free polyunsaturated margarine
1 tablespoon cornflour
1 tablespoon sugar
40mL (2 tablespoons) vinegar
250mL (1 cup) water

Saute pineapple, carrot and capsicum in margarine. Mix cornflour with a little water and add to pan. Combine sugar, vinegar and water. Gradually add to pan. Cook the sauce until thickened. (Serve with fish, chicken or pork.)

White Sauce

80g (4 tablespoons) polyunsaturated margarine
4 tablespoons cornflour
Pepper to taste
125mL (½ cup) cream
375mL (1½ cups) basic vegetable stock (page 17)

Melt margarine, add cornflour, pepper and cook until well blended. Mix cream and stock. Stir a little of this liquid into the cornflour mixture to form a smooth paste. Add the remaining liquid and cook until thickened. (Serve with fish or chicken.)

Brown Sauce

2 tablespoons polyunsaturated oil
80g (1 small) onion, diced
1½ tablespoons cornflour
300mL (1¼ cups) basic vegetable stock or water
2 teaspoons Worcestershire sauce
1 teaspoon vinegar
Pepper to taste

Heat oil and fry onion till brown. Remove from heat and add cornflour. Stir in stock or water to form a smooth paste. Return to heat and cook until sauce boils and thickens. Add Worcestershire sauce, vinegar and pepper, and simmer for 10 minutes.

Variations

MUSHROOM SAUCE   Add canned or chopped fresh mushrooms (approximately 50g) and simmer for 15 minutes.

SHERRY SAUCE   Add 2 tablespoons sherry and 2 tablespoons chopped parsley.

PIQUANT SAUCE   Add 1 tablespoon diced shallots.

Raisin Sauce

100g (½ cup) brown sugar
1 tablespoon cornflour
60g (¼ cup) seedless raisins
125mL (½ cup) vinegar
200mL (¾ cup) water

Combine sugar and cornflour in a saucepan. Add raisins, vinegar and water. Simmer over low heat to form a syrup.

Onion Sauce

480g (4 medium) onions, thinly sliced
80g (4 tablespoons) polyunsaturated margarine
1½ tablespoons cornflour
300mL (1¼ cups) water
½ teaspoon pepper

Fry onions in margarine until brown. Sprinkle with cornflour and stir in gently. Add water, pepper and simmer for 10 minutes. (Serve with pork or lamb chops.)

Creamy Salad Dressing

100mL (⅓ cup) cream
2 teaspoons vinegar
½ teaspoon mustard powder
½ teaspoon sugar
Pepper to taste

Combine all ingredients in a screw-top jar. Use within 2 to 3 days.

Variation

SEAFOOD SAUCE   Add 60mL (¼ cup) tomato sauce and 1 drop tabasco or Worcestershire sauce to cream dressing.

French Dressing

125mL (½ cup) polyunsaturated oil
60mL (¼ cup) vinegar
½ teaspoon dry mustard
½ teaspoon sugar
Pepper to taste
Small clove garlic, crushed (optional)

Place all ingredients in a screw-top jar and shake thoroughly until well blended. Store in the refrigerator.

Salads

These salads are based on vegetables and/or cereals. They can be substituted for a serving of bread, rice or pasta in your diet.

Rice Salad

SERVES 4

120g (½ cup) uncooked rice
40g (1 stick) celery, diced
30g (¼ cup) carrot, grated
60g (½ cup) capsicum, diced
100g (½ cup) pineapple, diced
¼ cup shallots, chopped

Dressing

40mL (2 tablespoons) polyunsaturated oil
40mL (2 tablespoons) vinegar
1 teaspoon French mustard
1 teaspoon sugar

Cook the rice in boiling, unsalted water. Drain and leave to cool. When the rice has cooled combine with celery, carrot, capsicum, pineapple and shallots.

Mix the dressing ingredients thoroughly and toss through the rice mixture.

Macaroni Salad

SERVES 10

160g (2 cups) uncooked macaroni
2 quantities creamy salad dressing (page 38)
60g (1 small) green capsicum
60g (1 small) red capsicum
150g mushrooms

180g (¾ cup) pineapple
¼ teaspoon ground pepper

Cook macaroni in boiling unsalted water. Rinse and drain thoroughly. Chop the capsicum, mushrooms and pineapple. In a large bowl combine cream dressing, pepper, capsicum, mushrooms and pineapple. Add the macaroni and toss well.

Tomato and Fettuccine Salad

SERVES 10

250g uncooked fettuccine
20mL (1 tablespoon) olive oil
2 tablespoons parsley, chopped
1 tablespoon chives, chopped
1 teaspoon tarragon
4 spring onion bulbs
80g (8) radishes
270g (2 medium) tomatoes
1 quantity French dressing (page 39)

Cook the fettuccine in boiling, unsalted water. Drain and place in a salad bowl with the oil, parsley, chives and tarragon. Combine gently. Cover and chill in refrigerator for at least 30 minutes. Chop the spring onion bulbs and radishes, and cut tomatoes into wedges. Before serving add the spring onions, radishes and french dressing. Toss well, then arrange tomato wedges around the bowl.

Tabouli

SERVES 10

225g (1½ cups) cracked wheat
1 bunch shallots, finely chopped
1½ cups chopped parsley
270g (2 medium) ripe tomatoes, finely chopped
80mL (⅓ cup) olive oil
60mL (¼ cup) fresh lemon juice

Soak cracked wheat in a bowl of water for 1 hour, then drain well. Mix in chopped shallots, parsley and tomatoes. Combine oil and lemon juice, add to salad and toss well.

Potato Salad

SERVES 4

360g (4 medium) potatoes
125mL (½ cup) cream
1 tablespoon white vinegar
2 tablespoons finely chopped onion
1 tablespoon finely chopped parsley

Boil potatoes until just tender, drain and allow to cool. Combine cream, white vinegar, onion and parsley. Dice the potatoes and fold into the cream mixture.

Fruit Desserts

These desserts are based on fruit and can be substituted for a serving of fruit in your diet.

Apricot Sago

SERVES 2

30g (3 tablespoons) uncooked sago
250mL (1 cup) apricot juice (from canned apricots)
2 tablespoons sugar
90g (8 halves) apricots, diced
2 tablespoons whipped cream

Soak sago in apricot juice for ½ hour. Cook gently until clear. Add sugar then cool. Place apricot pieces in 2 serving dishes. Add whipped cream to sago, stir in gently and pour over apricots. Chill before serving.

Lemon Sorbet

SERVES 4

250g (1 cup) sugar
600mL (2⅓ cups) water
1 tablespoon lemon rind
170mL (⅔ cup) fresh lemon juice

Dissolve sugar in water, bring to the boil and boil for about 15 minutes. Pour syrup over lemon rind and add lemon juice. Allow to cool. Strain and pour into freezing tray. Place in freezer. When half set, stir and return to freezer. Serve in chilled dessert glasses.

Variation
Add 200g pureed peaches along with the lemon juice.

Blancmange

SERVES 2

40g (¼ cup) cornflour
170mL (⅔ cup) undiluted cordial
300mL (1¼ cups) water
20g (1 tablespoon) polyunsaturated margarine

Mix cornflour to a smooth paste with the cordial. Add water and bring mixture to the boil, stirring constantly. Boil gently for 2 to 3 minutes. Add margarine. Pour into wetted moulds. Chill to set.

Lemon Cream

SERVES 4

2 tablespoons cornflour
60mL (3 tablespoons) lemon juice
170mL (⅔ cup) water
100g (½ cup) sugar
Grated rind of 1 lemon
1 drop yellow food colouring (optional)
1 tablespoon castor sugar
200mL (¾ cup) cream
Extra cream and lemon rind to decorate

Mix cornflour with lemon juice to form a smooth paste. Add water and sugar, place mixture over heat and bring to the boil. Remove from heat, add rind and colouring (if used). Cool completely without forming a skin. Add castor sugar to cream and whip until thick. Fold whipped cream into lemon mixture and place in serving glasses. Chill. Decorate with a little extra cream and lemon rind.

Banana Fritters

SERVES 2

60g (½ cup) cornflour
80mL (⅓ cup) water
200g (2 medium) bananas, peeled
Polyunsaturated oil, for frying
40g (2 tablespoons) castor sugar
½ teaspoon ground cinnamon

Blend cornflour with water. Cut bananas in half lengthwise and coat with the cornflour and water mixture. Fry in hot oil until golden brown. Roll in castor sugar and dust with cinnamon.

Baked Pineapple and Apples

SERVES 4

600g (4 medium) apples
20mL (1 tablespoon) fresh lemon juice
100g (½ cup) diced pineapple
3 tablespoons honey
Cinnamon
Nutmeg
Allspice
¼ cup water

Core apples and score skin around centre. Sprinkle with lemon juice. Fill centres of apples with pineapple and drizzle with honey. Place apples in an ovenproof dish and sprinkle with cinnamon, nutmeg and allspice. Add water to the bottom of the dish and bake in a hot oven (220C) for about 20 minutes or until tender, basting occasionally.

Serve hot or cold.

Variation
Substitute ½ cup berry fruit for pineapple

Bananas in Sherry

SERVES 4

600g (6 medium) firm bananas, peeled
45g (¼ cup firmly packed) brown sugar
125mL (½ cup) orange juice
Grated rind of 1 orange
¼ teaspoon cinnamon
¼ teaspoon nutmeg
75mL (¼ cup) sherry
30g (1½ tablespoons) salt-free polyunsaturated margarine

Place bananas in a greased baking dish. Combine sugar, juices, rind, spices and sherry. Heat and pour over bananas. Dot with margarine, cover and bake in a hot oven (240°C) for 10 to 15 minutes.

L'Orange au Grand Marnier

SERVES 6

900g (6 medium) oranges, peeled
200g (1 cup) castor sugar
60mL (3 tablespoons) Grand Marnier
6 tablespoons whipped cream to serve
6 twists orange rind to serve

Segment oranges and arrange them in a serving dish (1 orange per dish). Sprinkle with sugar and liqueur. Cover with foil and chill in the refrigerator for at least 12 hours. Decorate with whipped cream and a twist of orange rind before serving.

Apple and Lemon Dessert

SERVES 4

600g (4 medium) apples
60g (4 tablespoons) salt-free polyunsaturated margarine
50g (¼ cup) sugar
1 teaspoon lemon rind
40mL (2 tablespoons) fresh lemon juice

Peel, core and thinly slice the apples. Grease individual ramekins with margarine. Arrange alternate layers of apples, margarine, sugar and lemon rind. Finally, sprinkle a little lemon juice onto each ramekin. Cover with foil and bake in a medium oven (180°C) for 20 minutes.

Berry and Marshmallow Mousse

SERVES 4

375g canned berry fruit
60g (14 pieces) marshmallow
60mL (¼ cup) sherry
125mL (½ cup) cream, whipped

Drain the fruit and reserve syrup. Chop marshmallows and combine with sherry and reserved syrup. Fold in whipped cream. Arrange alternate layers of fruit and marshmallow mousse in dessert glasses. Chill before serving.

Creamy Desserts

These desserts contain slightly more protein and can be substituted for a serving of cereal, bread, rice or pasta in your diet.

Creamed Rice

SERVES 4

80g (⅓ cup) uncooked white rice
40g (2 tablespoons) sugar
1 teaspoon vanilla essence
20g (1 tablespoon) polyunsaturated margarine
125mL (½ cup) cream
Nutmeg or cinnamon to decorate

Cook rice in boiling, unsalted water until tender and drain. Add sugar, vanilla, margarine and mix well. Add cream and mix gently. Serve hot or cold, sprinkled with nutmeg or cinnamon.

Variation

Add 1 tablespoon sultanas.

Ice Cream

SERVES 4

100g (½ cup) sugar
30g (3 tablespoons) cornflour
300mL (1¼ cups) water
300mL (1¼ cups) cream
3 tablespoons vanilla essence

Mix sugar, cornflour and water in a saucepan. Stirring constantly, heat until the mixture boils and thickens. Remove from heat. Beat cream and vanilla essence in a small bowl until soft peaks form.

Pour in warm cornflour mixture in a thin stream. Combine gently. Semi-freeze mixture, then remove from freezer and whip until volume has increased. Semi-freeze again, whip and return to become cold.

Variations

* Add the pulp of 3 passionfruit into beaten mixture before freezing.
* Add 2 teaspoons of instant coffee or cocoa powder sifted with sugar.
* Fold 1 cup pureed fruit into beaten mixture before freezing.

Custard

SERVES 4

400mL (1¾ cups) cream
70g (⅓ cup) sugar
200mL (¾ cup) water
60g (½ cup) custard powder
Nutmeg to decorate

Heat cream, sugar and water in a saucepan, taking care not to boil. Blend some of this mixture into custard powder and add this back to the pan. Stir constantly over medium heat until the mixture has thickened. Serve sprinkled with a little nutmeg.

Sweet Sauces

These sauces contain small amounts of protein but up to 2 tablespoons per day can be used as an extra in your diet.

Orange and Lemon Sauce

125mL (½ cup) water
60g (3 tablespoons) sugar
Juice and finely grated rind of 1 lemon and 1 orange
1 tablespoon cornflour

Combine water, sugar, juices and rind. Bring to the boil. Blend cornflour with 1 tablespoon water and stir into sauce. Simmer, stirring for 1 minute.

Variation
Try adding some chopped ginger.

Orange Cinnamon Sauce

1 tablespoon cornflour
500mL (2 cups orange juice)
3 tablespoons honey
½ teaspoon cinnamon

Mix cornflour with a little orange juice and combine with remaining ingredients. Bring to the boil, stirring constantly.

Biscuits and Cakes

Two biscuits or 1 slice of cake can be exchange for a piece of bread in your diet.

Custard Kisses

MAKES 18

180g salt-free polyunsaturated margarine
60g (¼ cup) castor sugar
90g (⅔ cup) custard powder
125g (1 cup) cornflour
Jam of your choice

Cream margarine and sugar. Add sifted custard powder and cornflour. Roll into 36 balls. Flatten with a fork and place on greased baking sheets. Bake in a moderate oven (180°C) for 10–15 minutes until golden brown. Press two biscuits together with jam of your choice.

Honey Joys

MAKES 18

150g salt-free polyunsaturated margarine
120g (½ cup) sugar
220g (1 cup) honey
6 cups puffed rice

Combine margarine, sugar and honey in a pan and heat until sugar has dissolved. Add puffed rice and spoon into patty papers.

Corn Flake Biscuits

MAKES 12

40g (2 tablespoons) salt-free polyunsaturated margarine
1 tablespoon honey
2½ cups corn flakes

Melt margarine with honey until thin. Combine with corn flakes. Spoon into patty papers. Bake in a moderate oven (180°C) for 10 minutes.

Passionfruit Biscuits

MAKES 38

Biscuits

    250g (1 cup) salt-free polyunsaturated margarine
    90g (½ cup) icing sugar, sifted
    ½ cup passionfruit pulp (approximately 4 passionfruit)
    225g (1½ cups) self-raising flour
    125g (1 cup) cornflour

Icing

    120g (¾ cup) icing sugar, sifted
    1 teaspoon softened salt-free polyunsaturated margarine
    ¼ cup passionfruit pulp (approximately 2 passionfruit)

Cream margarine and icing sugar until light and fluffy. Add passionfruit pulp. Sift in flour. Flour hands, roll dough into 76 small balls and place on greased baking sheets. Flatten with a fork. Bake in a moderate oven (180°C) for 10 to 15 minutes. Allow to cool.

Combine icing sugar, margarine and enough passionfruit pulp to make a stiff paste. Sandwich 2 biscuits together with icing.

Melting Moment Biscuits

MAKES 16

170g salt-free polyunsaturated margarine
200g icing sugar
180g cornflour

Filling

1 tablespoon salt-free polyunsaturated margarine
50g pure icing sugar
2 teaspoons vanilla essence
300mL cream, whipped

Cream margarine and icing sugar. Add sifted cornflour and mix well. Roll into 32 small balls, place on greased baking sheets and flatten with a fork. Bake in a moderate oven (180°C) until golden brown, approximately 15 to 20 minutes.

Filling

Cream margarine. Add icing sugar, cream and vanilla essence. Add a little warm water if mixture needs softening. Sandwich biscuits with filling.

Carrot Cake

SERVES 10

150g (1 cup) self-raising wholemeal flour
Cinnamon
120g (½ cup) castor sugar
125mL polyunsaturated oil
75g (½ cup) honey
1 teaspoon vanilla essence
140g (1½ cups) finely grated carrot
100g (½ cup) sultanas or raisins

Combine all dry ingredients. Add oil and honey. Stir in vanilla essence, carrot and dried fruit. Spoon evenly into a greased and lined loaf tin and bake for 1 hour in moderate oven (180°C).

Apple Cake

SERVES 12

Apple Mixture

>450g (3 medium) apples, grated
>1 lemon rind, grated
>4 tablespoons sugar

Cake

>125g salt-free polyunsaturated margarine
>125g (½ cup) castor sugar
>2 × 60g eggs, lightly beaten
>180g (1½ cups) self-raising flour
>125g (1 cup) cornflour

Icing

>175g (1 cup) icing sugar, sifted
>2 tablespoons lemon juice (1 large lemon)
>1 teaspoon cinnamon

Combine all ingredients for apple mixture and set aside. Grease a lamington tin (base 19 × 29 cm). Cream margarine, sugar and eggs. Stir in lightly sifted flour, cornflour, then apple mixture. Bake in a moderate oven (180°C) for 30 minutes. Combine icing sugar and lemon juice. When cake is cool cover with icing and sprinkle with cinnamon.

Shortcrust Pastry

As this pastry recipe uses cornflour instead of wheat flour it does not increase the protein content of the final recipe.

>125g (1 cup) cornflour
>5g (1 teaspoon) baking powder
>50g (2½ tablespoons) salt-free polyunsaturated margarine
>50mL (2½ tablespoons) water

Sieve together dry ingredients. Rub margarine into flour until it resembles fine breadcrumbs. Add water and form a firm dough. Knead lightly and use as required.

Variation

For sweet pastry add 1½ tablespoons custard powder to cornflour.

CHAPTER

3

DIET AND RECIPES FOR THE PERSON ON HAEMODIALYSIS

The low-potassium diet	55
Fluid restriction	57
Eating out	58
Tips for watching your intake	63
Recipes	
Entrees	65
Main meals	69
Vegetables	80
Desserts	84
Cakes and biscuits	89

Once you commence dialysis, the machine will remove waste products and fluid from your body in place of your own kidneys. Since waste products, excess fluid and electrolytes can only be removed when you are on the machine, you may need to alter your food intake between dialysis treatments to prevent the build-up of excess waste. Whilst you may need to avoid or reduce your intake of certain foods, it is still important to eat the most nutritious diet possible.

Good nutrition is an important part of your treatment program.

THE LOW-POTASSIUM DIET

High blood levels of this mineral can cause paralysis of muscles, including the heart. This means that too much potassium could lead to a cardiac arrest. Potassium is found in almost all foods. It would be impossible to have a potassium-free diet but you should avoid those foods which are very high in potassium. Choose, where possible, the alternative which is lower in potassium.

Cook and prepare foods in the method which lowers the potassium content.

Foods Which are very High in Potassium

Dried fruits, bananas, rockmelon, figs, kiwi fruit, rhubarb, avocado, haricot beans, grapefruit, apricots, nectarines, paw paw, lentils, lima beans, soya beans, split peas, broad beans, chick peas, baked beans.

Nuts, potato crisps, liquorice, coconut, peanut butter, chocolate, soups.

Salt substitutes.

Choose the Alternative which is Lower in Potassium

Choose white rather than wholemeal bread. Choose refined cereals such as corn flakes and puffed rice, not wholegrain cereals such as muesli and bran flakes. Choose white rather than wholemeal rice and pasta.

Recently, much emphasis has been put on eating wholegrain foods because they are higher in dietary fibre and slightly higher in nutrients. However, white bread and refined cereals are not junk foods, they are still rich in nutrients, and are better for haemodialysis patients. It may be possible to include some wholegrain products in your diet to help relieve constipation.

Cooking to Lower the Potassium Content

Potassium readily dissolves in water. When a fruit or vegetable is boiled in water the potassium dissolves into the cooking water so that the cooked food is lower in potassium (do not consume the cooking water and juices).

In general, vegetables should be peeled, cut and soaked in a large volume of water before cooking. Stewed and canned fruit should be served without the juice or syrup. Stews and casseroles with lots of vegetables will be high in potassium, so try to drain off the gravy.

Sodium

You will find suggestions for flavouring foods without salt in the general introduction. Please note that some of these products are unsuitable for people who are also following a low-potassium diet. Many low-salt products now contain potassium chloride rather than sodium chloride.

Energy

The amount of energy in food is measured in kilojoules or calories. If you do not take enough energy you lose body weight. If you are losing body weight or have lost weight and cannot put it back on, you need to eat more energy-rich foods. The previous section on low-protein diets has some helpful hints. If you are overweight, you may need to decrease your energy intake.

Protein

Protein is made up of amino acids which are needed for the constant repair of body tissues. It is important that you eat enough protein but also important that you do not eat excessive amounts. Very high protein intakes lead to excessively high levels of urea in the blood which cannot be removed during the dialysis treatment. Your dietitian or doctor will have prescribed the appropriate amount of protein for you.

FLUID RESTRICTION

If you pass very little or no urine, the water you take in food and drink simply builds up in your body. The dialysis machine removes some water, but it cannot cope with unlimited amounts. Each one kilogram of weight you put on because of fluid build-up represents almost 1000mL (1 litre) of fluid. You should aim to keep your weight gain between dialysis treatments to a half kilogram per day.

The amount of fluid you can drink will depend on how much urine you pass and also how frequently and for how long you undergo dialysis. If you are gaining more than half a kilogram per day in between dialysis treatments then you need to cut back on your fluid intake. Beverages such as tea, coffee, water, soft drinks, cordial, milk and alcohol are obviously fluids. You will also need to keep a check on the fluid content of foods such as jelly (½ cup is 75mL fluid), ice cream (2 scoops is 50mL fluid), yoghurt (200g counts as 200mL), milk puddings (½ cup custard equals 125mL).

Helpful Hints for Fluid Control

1. If you avoid high-sodium foods, you will be less thirsty.
2. Try having allowed fruits and vegetables ice cold between meals.
3. Try a sliced lemon wedge to stimulate saliva and moisten a 'dry' mouth.
4. Use sour hard lollies and chewing gum to moisten mouth.
5. Rinse your mouth with water, but do not swallow it.
6. Remember ice is fluid but most people find ice more satisfying than the same amount of water, as it stays in the mouth longer.
7. Try putting lemon juice in ice cubes—you will use fewer. Use about half a lemon per tray of water.
8. Use very small cups and glasses for your drinks.
9. Try to keep yourself as active as possible. When you are idle, you may become preoccupied with a desire for liquids.
10. Be sure to eat well-balanced meals and you will have less desire for excess liquids.
11. If you use these guidelines and still gain too much weight, try keeping a liquids diary for a few days. Write down the exact quantities you are drinking throughout the day. You might be surprised at how quickly you use your fluid allowance.

EATING OUT

The following is a guide to best choices when eating out for haemodialysis patients.

Asian Cuisine

Best Choice

Omelettes	Sang Choy Bow
Prawn toasts	Curried prawns or chicken

Spring rolls
Dims Sims
Gow Gees
Garlic prawns
Chow Mein
Honey prawns

Steamed fish
Sweet and Sour
Boiled rice
Fried rice
Ice cream
Fortune cookies

Not Suitable

Soups
Soya sauce
Dishes with nuts or
   mushrooms or bamboo
   shoots

Satay sauce
Blackbean sauce
Coconut desserts
Lychees

Cafe, Cafeteria, Foodstand

Best Choice

Filled roll or sandwiches
   (white bread)
Toasted sandwiches
Cheese on toast
Hamburger
Steak sandwich
Hot dog
BBQ chicken
Sausage roll

Doughnuts
Scones
Cinnamon toast
Sponge cake
Pancakes with lemon
Ice cream (not chocolate)
Soft drinks
Tea/coffee
Capuccino/Vienna coffee

Not Suitable

Peanut butter
Vegemite
Soups
French fries
Potato scallops
Meat pies
Fruit buns/raisin bread
Chocolate cake

Fruit cake
Lamingtons
Cakes with nuts
Fruit salad
Fruit juices
Thickshakes
Milkshakes
Hot chocolate

French Cuisine

Best Choice

Pate
Frogs' legs
Quiche Lorraine
Savoury crepes
Grilled meat or fish
Steamed vegetables
Side salad
Bread

Garlic or herb bread
Creme caramel
Choux pastry with cream
Strawberries
Cheesecake
Ice cream
Croissant

Not Suitable

Soups
Rich sauces
Casseroles

French fries
Chocolate mousse
Profiteroles

Greek and Lebanese Cuisine

Best Choice

Yoghurt dip
Souvlaki
Mousaka
Doner kebab
Shish kebab
Grilled meat, chicken
Fish

Grilled octopus
Calamari
Boiled rice
Greek salad
Lebanese bread
Bread or bread rolls
Turkish delight

Not Suitable

Tahini
Hummus
Lady fingers
Spanakopita
Tabouli

Falafel
Kibbeh
Baklawa
Nougat

Italian Cuisine

Best Choice

Pasta with cream sauce
Veal in wine or lemon
Grilled fish or chicken
Salad
Bread/garlic bread

Vanilla ice cream
Lemon gelato
Strawberries
Italian torte

Not suitable

Minestrone
Pasta in tomato sauce
Dishes with spinach
Pizza

Profiteroles
Chocolate gelato
Cassata

Indian Cuisine

Best Choice

Meat, chicken or seafood curries
Tandoori chicken
Boiled rice

Cucumber raita
Roti
Papadams
Ice cream

Not Suitable

Bhayas
Vegetable curries
Dahl

Coconut desserts
Mango

International Cuisine

Best Choice

Prawn cocktail
Grilled seafood
Grilled meat
Grilled chicken

Pavlova
Cheesecake
Ice cream
Crepes

Grilled fish
Boiled vegetables

Apple pie
Cheese platter

Not Suitable

Soups
Avocado
Baked vegetables
Chips/French fries

Large amounts of sauce
Chocolate
Chocolate desserts
Fruit salad

Japanese Cuisine

Best Choice

Sushi/Sashimi
Tempura

Boiled rice

Not Suitable

Miso

Soya sauce

Mexican Cuisine

Best Choice

Tacos, burritos or enchiladas filled with meat or chicken
Grilled meat, chicken or seafood

Not Suitable

Tacos or burritos filled with beans
Nachos
Guacamole

Frijoles
Fruitcake

Seafood

Best Choice

Oysters, prawns
Grilled scallops or octopus

Salad
Bread/garlic or herb bread

Calamari
Seafood crepes
Grilled or fried fish
Seafood platter
Steamed vegetables

Ice cream
Strawberries
Pavlova
Cheesecake
Cheese platter

Not Suitable

Soup
Chowder
Chips
French fries

Chocolate cakes
Chocolate desserts
Fruit salad

Vegetarian Cuisine

Best Choice

Steamed vegetables
Vegetable strudel
Rice
Pasta

Egg dishes
Crepes
Vol-au-vent
Cheese platter

Not Suitable

Soups
Dishes with dried beans and lentils
Nuts

Banana Cake
Cakes and desserts with fruit or nuts.

TIPS FOR WATCHING YOUR INTAKE

Sodium and Potassium

A number of foods listed as best choices, whilst low in potassium, will be high in salt. If you are eating these foods on an occasional basis only then this is acceptable.

In general, avoid soups, avocado and fruit starters. Select grills or pan-fried meat, chicken, fish and seafood rather than dishes with rich sauces and gravies. Avoid chips and roast vegetables and ask for boiled or steamed vegetables without salt and sauce. Avoid chocolate-based desserts, fruit salad and sweets with dried fruit and nuts.

Avoid most unlabelled commercially prepared foods as the protein and sodium levels can be both high and variable, e.g. savoury tinned food, sausage rolls, frozen packet meals.

Fluids

Try to drink less throughout the day if you wish to drink more with a special meal out. Beware of having your glass topped up, as this makes it difficult to estimate how much you are drinking. Do not forget to make allowance for fruit, jellies or milk puddings as these all contain fluid. No more than two standard alcoholic drinks per day are advised.

Remember, the important thing is to keep to your fluid restriction.

Entrees

Vegetable Lasagne

SERVES 10

200g (1 packet) uncooked or precooked lasagne noodles
20mL (1 tablespoon) water
240g (2 medium) onions
2 cloves garlic, crushed
405g (3 medium) tomatoes, chopped
1 tablespoon dried or 2 tablespoon chopped fresh oregano
½ tablespoon dried or 1 tablespoon chopped fresh basil
3 tablespoons fresh parsley, chopped
500mL (2 cups) low-protein white sauce
1 teaspoon paprika

Cook lasagne noodles in boiling, unsalted water, then cover with cold water to prevent further cooking and set aside. (If using precooked lasagne noodles omit this step.)

Heat the water or use a non-stick large frying pan to saute onion and garlic until soft. Add tomatoes and herbs. Cook for 25 to 30 minutes until mixture has thickened. Prepare white sauce (see below). Preheat oven to 180°C.

To assemble, place a layer of lasagne noodles in baking dish, cover with a third of the quantity of tomato sauce and then white sauce. Repeat layers, finishing with white sauce. Sprinkle with paprika. Bake for 30 minutes, remove from oven and allow 15 minutes before serving.

Low-Protein White Sauce

20g (1 tablespoon) polyunsaturated salt-free margarine
20g (2 tablespoons) cornflour
440mL (1¾ cups) water
125mL (½ cup) cream

Melt margarine, add cornflour and stir well. Allow to simmer for 2 minutes. Slowly add water and cream, stirring constantly, until boiled and thickened.

Red Capsicum Relish Rolls

SERVES 8

100g (½ cup) uncooked white rice
80g (1 medium) red capsicum
240g (2 medium) onions, finely chopped
2 cloves garlic, crushed
1 teaspoon mustard seeds
½ teaspoon dried (or 1 teaspoon fresh chopped) basil
20mL (1 tablespoon) polyunsaturated oil
405g (3 medium) tomatoes, diced
½ teaspoon curry powder
50g (2 tablespoons) brown sugar
40mL (2 tablespoons) vinegar
8 sheets filo pastry
Polyunsaturated oil for brushing

Cook rice in boiling, unsalted water. Remove seeds and membrane from capsicum and cut into fine strips. Fry capsicum, onion, garlic, mustard seeds and basil in oil. Add tomatoes and curry powder. Cover and allow to cook for a few minutes. Add sugar and vinegar, cook and stir. Remove from heat, stir in cooked white rice. Leave for 5 minutes then stir again. Fold one sheet of filo pastry in half, add 2 tablespoons of mixture to end of pastry and roll half way. Fold in sides and roll all the way to the end. Repeat assembling rolls in same manner with remaining pastry. Brush a baking tray with oil and lay filo rolls in tray about 2cm apart. Brush with oil and bake in a moderate oven (180°C) till brown, approximately 30 minutes.

Mustard and Potato Spring Rolls

SERVES 6

180g (2 medium) potatoes
5g (1 teaspoon) mustard seeds
50g (½ cup) mung bean sprouts
120g (1 medium) onion, thinly sliced
½ teaspoon fennel seeds
½ clove garlic, crushed
1 tablespoon chives, chopped
30g (1 tablespoon) salt-free polyunsaturated margarine
12 sheets spring roll wrappers

Dressing

    125g (½ cup) sour cream
    1 tablespoon french mustard
    5mL (1 teaspoon) lemon juice
    2 teaspoons chives, chopped

Scrub, dice and soak potatoes in water for 2 hours. Discard water. Cook in fresh water and drain on absorbent kitchen paper. Lightly pan-fry mustard seeds, mung bean sprouts, onion, fennel seeds, garlic and chives in margarine. Stir-fry for approximately 2 minutes. Stir in potato. Spoon into spring roll sheets and fold up in envelope fashion. Deep fry until golden brown.

Mix together all dressing ingredients. Serve spring rolls hot, dipped in the dressing.

Broccoli and Pea Vol-Au-Vents

SERVES 8

    120g broccoli, cut into flowerettes
    70g (½ cup) peas
    30g (1½ tablespoons) salt-free polyunsaturated margarine
    20g (1½ tablespoons) white flour
    170mL (⅔ cup) cream
    40mL (2 tablespooon) dry white wine
    1 tablespoon chives, chopped
    8 large vol-au-vent cases (or 16 small)
    Pepper
    Paprika
    Chives, chopped
    Lemon wedges

Soak broccoli and peas in water for 2 hours, then discard the water. Boil in fresh water till cooked. Melt margarine in a saucepan and remove from heat. Stir in flour and blend in cream, wine and chives. Bring to the boil while stirring, add broccoli and peas and simmer mixture for 2 to 3 minutes. Heat vol-au-vent cases in a moderate oven (180°C) for a few minutes till crisp and hot. Fill cases with hot mixture, sprinkle with paprika, pepper, chives and decorate with small lemon wedges.

Eggplant and Ginger Rolls

SERVES 8

100g (½ cup) uncooked white rice
500g eggplant, cubed
240g (2 medium) onions, finely chopped
20mL (1 tablespoon) polyunsaturated oil
2 teaspoons seed mustard
1 tablespoon fresh ginger, finely diced
8 sheets filo pastry
Polyunsaturated oil for brushing

Cook rice in boiling, unsalted water. Soak eggplant in water for one hour and drain well. Saute eggplant and onion in oil. Mix in mustard, ginger and rice. Fold one sheet of filo pastry in half. Add 2 tablespoons of mixture to the edge of the sheet. Roll pastry half way, then fold in the sides and roll to the end of pastry. Repeat, assembling rolls in same manner with remaining pastry. Grease a baking tray with oil, lay filo rolls in the tray about 2cm apart. Brush with oil. Bake in moderate oven (180°C) until brown, approximately 30 minutes.

Main Meals

Chicken Chinese Style

SERVES 6

500g chicken breast fillets
1 egg white
20mL (1 tablespoon) dry sherry
10g (1 tablespoon) cornflour
60g (1 small) red capsicum
60g (1 small) green capsicum
80mL (4 tablespoons) polyunsaturated oil
Slice of fresh ginger
1 clove garlic, crushed
Few drops sesame oil

Seasoning

20mL (1 tablespoon) dry sherry
1 teaspoon sugar
2 teaspoons salt-reduced soya sauce
1 teaspoon cornflour
60mL (¼ cup) salt-free chicken stock or water

Remove skin and bones from chicken. Cut flesh into 2.5cm cubes and place in a bowl with egg white, sherry and cornflour. Stir with a fork or chopsticks until well combined. Halve capsicums, deseed and cut into 2.5cm squares. Mix all seasoning ingredients in a small bowl. Heat 3 tablespoons of oil in a wok or frypan and add ginger and crushed garlic. Discard ginger when it begins to colour. Add a few drops of sesame oil then add chicken and stir over high heat until it begins to colour. Remove to a plate. Add remaining oil to frypan and fry capsicum for two minutes. Return chicken, stir well and add seasoning mix. Stir until mixture boils. Serve immediately on a bed of boiled white rice.

HEALTHY EATING ON A RENAL DIET

Chicken Marengo

SERVES 4

350g (4) chicken thigh fillets
Pepper
40mL (2 tablespoons) polyunsaturated oil
30g (1½ tablespoons) polyunsaturated salt-free margarine
12 small mushrooms
250mL (1 cup) water
1 clove garlic, crushed
1 teaspoon cornflour
270g (2 medium) ripe tomatoes, skinned, deseeded and chopped
1 teaspoon oregano
125mL (½ cup) dry white wine
20g (1 tablespoon) salt-free tomato paste

Sprinkle chicken fillets with pepper. Saute chicken in a large frypan with oil and margarine. Brown on all sides till almost cooked. Remove chicken and keep warm. In a small saucepan, simmer mushrooms in water, drain and reserve liquid. Add garlic and flour to the juices left in frypan and stir over a low heat for 1 minute. Add tomatoes and oregano. Simmer for a few minutes, then add wine and ½ cup of the mushroom liquid. Bring to boil, reduce heat and simmer uncovered for 15 minutes. Add tomato paste. Return chicken pieces to pan, add mushrooms and simmer all together for 5 minutes. Serve with boiled white rice or noodles.

Cannelloni

SERVES 6

120g (1 medium) onion, finely chopped
160g (2 medium) carrots, grated
120g (2 small) zucchini, grated
80mL (⅓ cup) polyunsaturated oil
1 clove garlic, crushed
2 teaspoon fresh parsley, chopped

150g mince meat
20g (1 tablespoon) plain white flour
625mL (2½ cups) water
Pinch oregano
Pinch basil
Pinch nutmeg
Pinch pepper
60g (⅔ cup) breadcrumbs
60g (3 tablespoons) cottage cheese
1 × 55g egg
12 cannelloni cases, instant precooked variety
250mL (1 cup) white sauce
Extra nutmeg

Soak onions, carrot and zucchini in separate containers of water for 2 hours. Drain and discard water. In a saucepan, brown onions in oil, add garlic, parsley, carrot and zucchini. Add mince and brown. Stir in flour and add water slowly while stirring. Add oregano, basil, nutmeg and pepper and allow to boil for about 15 minutes or until mixture is thick. Allow to cool. Add breadcrumbs, cottage cheese, egg and mix well. Make the white sauce (see below).

To assemble, stuff each cannelloni shell with 3 tablespoon of mixture. Place in a greased casserole dish. Pour white sauce over the cannelloni. Sprinkle with a little nutmeg. Bake in a moderate oven (180°C) for 40 minutes or until golden brown.

White Sauce

40g (2 tablespoons) polyunsaturated salt-free margarine
40g (2 tablespoons) plain white flour
125mL (½ cup) milk
125mL (½ cup) cream
1 tablespoon parsley, chopped

Melt margarine in a saucepan. Add flour and stir until well combined. Cook for one minute. Add milk in a steady stream, stirring constantly. Sauce will begin to thicken. Add cream and parsley and stir well.

Beef Fillets with Tarragon Wine Sauce

SERVES 8

30g (1½ tablespoons) polyunsaturated salt-free margarine
700g beef eye fillet, in one piece
500mL (2 cups) dry white wine
30g (1½ tablespoons) polyunsaturated salt-free margarine (extra)
4 green shallots, chopped finely
20g (1 tablespoon) plain white flour
1 teaspoon dried tarragon leaves, crushed
125mL (½ cup) water
20mL (1 tablespoon) cream
Lemon slices to garnish

Melt margarine in pan, add beef and cook over high heat, turning meat until browned all over. Transfer beef to an ovenproof dish and bake in a moderate oven for 25 minutes or until beef is done as desired. Stand 5 minutes before slicing.

Meanwhile, add wine to pan juices, simmer until liquid is reduced to half and pour into a jug. Melt extra margarine in pan, add shallots, stir in flour and tarragon. Gradually blend in the wine mixture. Add water and cream, stir over low heat until sauce begins to boil and thicken. Serve over the sliced beef. Garnish with lemon slices.

Garlic Lamb Chops

SERVES 6

6 × 60g lamb loin chops
Pepper
10mL (2 teaspoons) polyunsaturated oil
10mL (2 teaspoons) polyunsaturated salt-free margarine
2–3 cloves garlic, crushed
1 teaspoon thyme
60mL (¼ cup) water
Fresh thyme (optional)

Sprinkle chops with pepper. In a frypan, brown chops in polyunsaturated oil. Remove from pan and set aside. Pour oil off from pan, add margarine, garlic and thyme. Reduce heat and cook for 3 minutes. Add chops and water, increase heat and immediately cover the pan. When the juices are bubbling serve at once accompanied by vegetables and garnished with a sprig of fresh thyme.

Veal Scallopini

SERVES 8

225g mushrooms, sliced
70g (3½ tablespoons) polyunsaturated salt-free margarine
30mL (1½ tablespoons) lemon juice
480g veal, cut into thin slices
Pepper
50g (2 tablespoons) brown sugar
Plain white flour for seasoning
180mL (¾ cup) dry white wine
1 tablespoon parsley, chopped

Saute mushrooms in 2 tablespoons of margarine until just tender. Sprinkle with lemon juice and set aside. Cut veal into 2.5cm strips. Sprinkle with pepper and brown sugar. Dip veal strips in flour. Melt remainder of margarine in a frypan. Add wine and cook rapidly for a few minutes. Add mushrooms, heat thoroughly. Sprinkle with parsley and serve on a bed of rice.

Veal Paprika

SERVES 5

300g veal
60mL (3 tablespoons) polyunsaturated oil
320g (4 small) onions, quartered
1 clove garlic, crushed
40g (2 tablespoons) salt-free tomato paste
250mL (1 cup) water
125mL (½ cup) dry red wine
1 teaspoon paprika
Pepper to taste

Cut veal into 2.5cm cubes. In a large frypan, heat oil over medium heat. Brown veal on all sides. Remove veal from frypan and set aside. Add onion and garlic to pan and cook, stirring constantly, for 2 minutes. Stir in tomato paste, loosen pan juices by stirring bottom of pan well. Add veal, water, wine, paprika and pepper. Cover and stir occasionally. Cook for 30 minutes or until veal is tender.

Veal Birds

SERVES 10

700g veal steak
English mustard
Plain flour
Pepper
Polyunsaturated oil for frying
125mL (½ cup) salt-free stock or water
Parsley and whole peppercorns to garnish

Stuffing

100g (1 cup) soft white breadcrumbs
½ teaspoon mixed herbs
½ beaten egg (or 1 egg yolk)
Pepper

Thinly slice veal into 10 even rectangular pieces and pound. Mince any trimmings and add to stuffing. Lightly spread veal with very little mustard. Mix stuffing ingredients together. Spread stuffing on veal, roll and secure with a toothpick or string. Roll in flour seasoned with pepper and brown in a little hot oil. Place in a casserole dish and add stock or water. Cover dish and cook slowly in the centre of a moderate oven (180°C) for about 45 to 60 minutes. Serve with rice and garnish with parsley and whole peppercorns.

Apple and Pork Chop Roast

SERVES 6

180g (2 small) apples
125mL (½ cup) white wine
60mL (¼ cup) lemon juice
¼ teaspoon dry mustard
40mL (2 tablespoons) polyunsaturated oil
6 × 60g pork rib chops
1 teaspoon cumin
1 teaspoon thyme
1 teaspoon basil
Pepper to taste

Core and peel apples. Cut into thin slices. Preheat oven to 180°C. Mix wine, lemon juice, dry mustard and oil together, brush onto chops and reserve remainder for basting. Season chops with herbs and pepper. Alternate pork chops and apple slices to form the shape of a roast. Secure with wooden skewers. Place in an ungreased baking tray. Bake, uncovered, for 15 minutes. Reduce temperature to low (120°C) and bake for a further 50 minutes, basting occasionally.

Turkey Fillets in Sour Cream

SERVES 8

500g turkey breast fillets
Fine breadcrumbs
Pepper
Mixed herbs
2 × 60g eggs
40mL (2 tablespoons) water
Salt-free polyunsaturated margarine for frying
1 tablespoon onion, finely chopped
1 tablespoon paprika
1 tablespoon paprika
2 tablespoons shallots, chopped
300mL (1¼ cups) sour cream
20g (1 tablespoon) plain flour
Chopped shallots to garnish

Cut turkey fillets into 8 uniform pieces. Season breadcrumbs with pepper and mixed herbs. Beat eggs and water together. Dip turkey pieces in seasoned breadcrumbs then in beaten egg and finally dip again in breadcrumbs. Brown fillets on both sides in hot margarine and transfer to a baking dish. Sprinkle with onions and parsley. Add ¼ cup water. Pour sour cream over fillets, sprinkle with paprika, cover dish and bake in a moderate oven (180°C) for 15 minutes. Reduce heat to 120°C and bake for a further 30 minutes or until tender. Remove cover and increase heat for the last few minutes of cooking to crisp coating. Transfer turkey to a heated platter. Transfer sauce to a small saucepan, heat and stir in flour. Cook till thickened. Pour over turkey and serve hot, garnished with chopped shallots.

Lemon Sesame Chicken

SERVES 7

10mL (2 teaspoons) polyunsaturated oil
10mL (2 teaspoons) polyunsaturated salt-free margarine
425g chicken thigh fillets, sliced
30mL (1½ tablespoons) lemon juice
Pinch of rosemary leaves
Pinch of thyme
Pinch of marjoram
2 teaspoons of sesame seeds
Pepper to taste
45g (1½ tablespoons) honey
1 tablespoon cornflour
30mL (1½ tablespoons) water
Parsley and lemon slices to garnish

Preheat oven to 180°C. In a frypan, heat oil and margarine and fry chicken fillets for 10 minutes, turning to brown. Arrange chicken in a lightly greased baking dish. Mix remaining ingredients and brush half of mixture over chicken. Bake, uncovered for 1 hour, brushing frequently with remaining mixture. Garnish with a sprig of parsley and lemon slices.

Hungarian Goulash

SERVES 10

40g (2 tablespoons) polyunsaturated salt-free margarine
30mL (1½ tablespoons) oil
800g stewing steak, cut into cubes
480g (4 medium) onions, sliced
1 clove garlic, crushed
1½ tablespoons paprika
½ teaspoon black pepper
160mL (⅔ cup) water
1 bay leaf
125mL (½ cup) sour cream

Heat margarine and oil in a large saucepan using a moderate heat. Add cubes of steak a few at a time and brown on all sides. Remove from pan and set aside. Add onions to saucepan. Cook for 8 to 10 minutes or until golden brown. Add garlic, paprika and pepper. Then add steak, water and bay leaf and stir well. When mixture comes to the boil, put saucepan lid on, reduce heat and allow to simmer for 2 hours. Taste and add more pepper if necessary. Remove bay leaf and discard. Stir in sour cream. Serve hot over rice or noodles. Garnish with parsley leaves.

Fillets of Fish with Zucchini

SERVES 4

135g (1 medium) tomato
170g (3 medium) zucchini
20mL (1 tablespoon) polyunsaturated oil
1 sprig of rosemary
1 teaspoon fresh, chopped basil
Pepper
30g (2 tablespoons) plain white flour
440g (4) fish fillets, eg. sole, barramundi, whiting or dory
80g (4 tablespoons) salt-free polyunsaturated margarine
100g (1 cup) dry breadcrumbs
12 basil leaves
1 lemon, sliced

Peel and chop the tomato and slice the zuccini. Saute zucchini in oil and add rosemary, basil and pepper. When nearly cooked add tomatoes and saute for a further 2 minutes. Flour fish fillets and fry until brown in 3 tablespoons of margarine. Grease an ovenproof dish and arrange fillets in a row. Cover with zucchini mixture, sprinkle with breadcrumbs, dot with remaining margarine and bake in a hot oven (220°C) for a few minutes till brown. Serve with basil leaves and lemon slices.

Fish Cakes

SERVES 6

315g redfish fillets
315g mashed potato
20g (1 tablespoon) polyunsaturated salt-free margarine
2 × 60g eggs
3 teaspoons plain white flour
¼ teaspoon cayenne pepper
6 teaspoons fresh parsley, chopped
125g (1 cup) fine dry breadcrumbs
60mL (¼ cup) polyunsaturated oil

Cook, skin and flake the fish. In a large mixing bowl combine fish, potato, margarine, 1 egg, flour, cayenne pepper and parsley. Mix well with a wooden spoon. Place in refrigerator to chill for 1 hour. With floured hands, shape mixture into about 6 balls. On a lightly floured board, flatten to patties. Beat the remaining egg, then dip patties into beaten egg and roll in breadcrumbs. In a large frypan, heat oil over high heat and add fish cakes. Fry for 5 to 8 minutes, turning frequently until golden brown. Serve with bread and vegetables.

Fish Rolls

SERVES 4

500g (4) fish fillets
10g (½ tablespoon) polyunsaturated salt-free margarine
50g (¼ cup) onion, finely chopped
60g (¼ cup) celery, finely chopped
100g (½ cup) mushrooms, sliced
4 tablespoon parsley, chopped
40mL (2 tablespoons) lemon juice
Pepper

Remove bones from fish fillets. Heat margarine in a pan and saute onion and celery until tender. Add mushrooms, parsley and lemon juice. Divide mixture evenly between the fillets and spread over each fillet. Roll up each fillet and secure with a toothpick. Place in a lightly greased baking tray. Bake in a moderate oven (180°C) for 20 to 25 minutes.

Peppered Calamari

SERVES 5

500g calamari rings
1 tablespoon cracked pepper
20mL (1 tablespoon) polyunsaturated oil

Marinade

250mL (1 cup) port or red wine
125mL (1 cup) olive oil
80g (1 small) onion, sliced roughly
4 cloves garlic, crushed
3 bay leaves

In a bowl combine all marinade ingredients. Mix well. Place calamari rings in the marinade and allow to stand overnight. Drain calamari and sprinkle with black pepper. Brush a barbeque plate with oil and cook calamari on hotplate for 30 seconds. Alternatively, the calamari may be cooked in a frypan. Serve with crusty bread.

Vegetables

Scalloped Potatoes

SERVES 10

270g (3 medium) potatoes
120g (1 medium) onion
180mL (⅔ cup) cream
35g (⅓ cup) dry breadcrumbs
2 teaspoons paprika
¼ teaspoon pepper

Peel, wash and slice potatoes. Soak for 2 hours in water and discard water. Steam the potato slices for 5 minutes. Slice onion thinly. Arrange potatoes and onions in alternate layers in a baking dish. Pour cream over. Mix paprika with breadcrumbs and pepper and sprinkle over top. Bake in a moderate oven (180°C) for 1 hour.

Caramelized Carrots

SERVES 4

320g (4 medium) carrots
20g (1 tablespoon) brown sugar
30g (1½ tablespoons) salt-free polyunsaturated margarine

Peel, wash and thickly slice carrots. Soak in water for 2 hours and discard water. Cook carrots in a small amount of fresh water until water has reduced to about 3mm in the bottom of the saucepan. Add sugar and margarine. Toss carrots until the sugar is dissolved.

Gingered Beetroot

SERVES 4

360g (4 medium) beetroots
70g (⅓ cup) brown sugar

¾ teaspoon ground ginger
5g (2 teaspoons) cornflour
20mL (1 tablespoon) cider vinegar
20g (1 tablespoon) polyunsaturated salt-free margarine
1 tablespoon fresh parsley, chopped

Wash beetroot, soak in water for 2 hours and discard water. Boil beetroot in its skin in fresh water for 30 minutes. Peel and slice. In a saucepan blend sugar, ginger and cornflour together. Gradually add vinegar, stirring over heat until smooth and thickened. Add beetroot slices and margarine, simmer 5 minutes longer. Serve piping hot, sprinkled with chopped parsley.

Broccoli Florentine

SERVES 8

500g broccoli
3 cloves garlic, crushed
60mL (¼ cup) polyunsaturated oil
Ground black pepper

Trim tough ends from broccoli. Peel stems and make 2 slits crosswise in base of stems to speed cooking. Soak broccoli in water for 2 hours and discard water. Stand broccoli upright in a saucepan containing a little boiling water. Cover and cook until stems are just tender (12 to 15 minutes). Drain and cut broccoli into large pieces. Fry crushed garlic in oil. As garlic browns, add broccoli and saute until tender, turning pieces frequently. Season with freshly ground pepper.

Green Beans Oregano

SERVES 4

260g green beans
2 teaspoons dried or 1 tablespoon fresh oregano
20g (1 tablespoon) salt-free polyunsaturated margarine
Sprig of oregano or parsley to garnish

Soak beans for 2 hours in water and discard water. Cook beans and oregano together in fresh boiling water, drain and toss in margarine before serving. Garnish with fresh oregano or parsley.

Spicy Fried Corn

SERVES 4

160g (1 cup) corn kernels
8g (1½ teaspoons) salt-free polyunsaturated margarine
1 teaspoon finely chopped onion
1 teaspoon paprika
Pepper
1 tablespoon parsley, chopped

Soak corn for 2 hours in water and discard water. Cook corn in fresh boiling water. Drain well. Melt margarine in a small saucepan, stir in cooked corn and onion. Saute for about 2 minutes over heat. Add paprika, pepper and cook for an additional 2 to 3 minutes. Sprinkle with chopped parsley.

Pineapple and Capsicum Coleslaw

SERVES 6

500g raw cabbage
60g (1 small) green capsicum
250mL (1 cup) crushed sweetened pineapple, drained
40g (2 tablespoons) polyunsaturated salt-reduced mayonnaise
30g (1½ tablespoons) cider vinegar
¼ teaspoon dill seeds
Pepper

Finely shred the cabbage. Remove seeds and membrane from the capsicum and chop finely. Soak cabbage and capsicum in water for 2 hours. Discard water and drain well. Combine cabbage, capsicum and pineapple. Mix mayonnaise, vinegar, dill seed and pepper. Pour over vegetables and toss. Cover and refrigerate for 1 to 2 hours before serving.

Old-fashioned Macaroni Salad

SERVES 6

250g (1 cup) uncooked elbow-shaped macaroni
1 × 55g egg
30g (½ small) green capsicum
65g (¼ cup) polyunsaturated salt-reduced mayonnaise
20g (1 tablespoon) sour cream
30mL (1½ tablespoons) cider vinegar
½ teaspoon dry mustard
Pepper
2 tablespoons finely chopped parsley
Orange slices to garnish

Cook macaroni in boiling, unsalted water. Drain and refrigerate. Hard boil, then peel and chop the egg. Deseed the capsicum and chop into small squares. In a large bowl beat mayonnaise, sour cream, vinegar, mustard and pepper until smooth. Mix in macaroni, chopped egg and chopped capsicum. Sprinkle with finely chopped parsley. Refrigerate before serving. Decorate with sliced orange.

Desserts

Biscotten Torte (Almond Torte)

SERVES 8

75mL milk
40mL (2 tablespoons) brandy
1 packet morning coffee biscuits
125g (½ cup) salt-free polyunsaturated margarine
120g (½ cup) castor sugar
12 Sao biscuits, crushed
2 × 55g eggs
1 teaspoon almond essence
75mL milk
300mL cream, whipped

Mix milk and brandy together in a bowl. Dip biscuits into this mixture, just enough to moisten well. Lay biscuits on a flat serving dish, two biscuits wide and four long.

To make the filling, cream margarine and sugar. Add egg yolks. Beat again, adding Sao crumbs, almond essence and milk. Beat egg whites until slightly stiff and combine with the above mixture.

Spread one-quarter of the filling on top of biscuit layer. Cover with another layer of biscuits and repeat this process until all the filling is used. The top layer is biscuit. Cover the torte with plastic or foil wrap. Refrigerate for 24 hours or freeze for several hours.

Before serving, cover the torte with whipped cream. If desired, torte may be decorated with crushed toffee, cinnamon or nutmeg.

Bandeux Aux Fruits

SERVES 16

375g frozen puff pastry
20g (1) egg yolk
10g (1 tablespoon) castor sugar

Filling

3 × 55g eggs
50g (¼ cup) castor sugar
20g (2 tablespoons) cornflour
125mL (½ cup) milk
Vanilla essence

Decoration

8 canned peach slices, well drained
4 canned cherries, well drained
2 canned pineapple rings, well drained
Whipped cream

Grease an 8 × 26cm bar tin and line with foil. Roll out pastry into a rectangle about 30 × 12cm. Cut off 2 strips from the end and from the sides about 2cm in width. These will form the edges of the base. Line prepared tin with pastry. Brush the base pastry with the egg yolk beaten with sugar. Attach the edges to the base and bake in a hot oven (220°C) until the pastry rises and is golden brown (approximately 15 minutes). Allow pastry to cool.

In a bowl, mix eggs and sugar together, then add cornflour and enough milk to form a smooth paste. In a saucepan, boil the remainder of the milk. Add hot milk to the egg mixture, stirring constantly to prevent lumps forming. Return mixture to saucepan, place on hotplate and allow mixture to cook and thicken whilst stirring. Spread custard into the pastry case. Arrange fruit on top of custard. Refrigerate for several hours before serving. To serve, slice and decorate with piped cream.

Strawberry Meringue Flan

SERVES 8

    4 egg whites
    220g (1 cup) castor sugar

Filling

    500g (2 punnets) strawberries
    250mL (1 cup) cream
    40g (2 tablespoons) castor sugar
    Vanilla essence

Oil a large pavlova tray and line with greaseproof paper or aluminium foil. Beat egg whites in a small bowl with electric mixer until they form soft peaks. Continue to beat, adding a little sugar at a time, until all the sugar has been added. Spread ¾ of the mixture into a circle with a spatula on the pavlova tray and then pipe the remaining mixture around the edge of the circle to build up the sides. Bake at 120°C on the lowest shelf of the oven until the meringue is completely dried out (approximately 2 hours). When meringue is crisp, remove from the oven and allow to cool.

Wash the strawberries and remove stalks. Whip the cream, castor sugar and a few drops of vanilla essence together. Spread the inside of the flan with the cream and then place strawberries on the top.

Crème Brulée

SERVES 4

    4 egg yolks
    60g (¼ cup) castor sugar
    500mL (2 cups) cream
    Vanilla essence

Caramel topping

    100g (½ cup) sugar
    60mL (¼ cup water)

Blend together egg yolks and sugar. Add cream to the egg mixture and stir in a few drops of vanilla essence. Strain mixture into 4 medium-sized ramekins. Stand ramekins in a baking tray containing 2.5cm of hot water. Bake custard until firm in a cool oven (120°C). This takes approximately 45 minutes. Leave in the refrigerator overnight.

Next day, make the caramel topping. Dissolve sugar and water over a low heat and then boil rapidly until a pale caramel colour. Quickly pour three-quarters of the caramel over the tops of the chilled custard. Leave the remainder of the caramel to set on a well-oiled tray. When set, crush and use to decorate the edges of the dishes.

Honey and Apple Crepe Gateau

SERVES 4

150g (1 cup) plain white flour
15g (3 teaspoons) sugar
3 egg yolks
75g (⅓ cup) salt-free polyunsaturated margarine, melted
190mL (¾ cup) milk
190mL (¾ cup) cold water
Polyunsaturated oil for cooking

Filling

500g (4 medium) green cooking apples
½ lemon
Ground cinnamon
Castor sugar
Honey
Extra cinnamon and castor sugar
Whipped cream
Slices of lemon to garnish

Sift flour into a mixing bowl and stir in the sugar. Beat in the egg yolks, margarine, and milk. Gradually beat in the cold water. Continue to beat until a smooth batter is achieved.

Lightly grease a crepe pan with some polyunsaturated oil. Pour a thin layer of crepe batter into the pan and rotate the pan so that the batter is evenly distributed. Cook about one minute or until crepe is brown. Turn and cook on other side for about 30 seconds. Slide the crepe out of the pan. Repeat until all the batter is cooked.

Filling

Peel and core apples, cut into thick slices. Soak in cold water for two hours, discard water and drain well. Grate the lemon rind and add to the apples with the juice of the lemon. Cook on a low heat in a heavy saucepan and allow apples to soften. Stir occasionally to prevent sticking. When soft, beat with a wooden spoon, adding a pinch of cinnamon and, if too tart, sweeten with castor sugar.

To Serve

Spread one crepe with a little honey and then apple mixture. Transfer this to a round, ovenproof dish and continue to add layers in the same way on top of the first crepe. End with an uncovered crepe. Sprinkle with a little extra cinnamon mixed with castor sugar and heat in a slow oven (120°C) for 10 to 15 minutes. To serve, cut through the layers like a cake and decorate each slice with whipped cream. Garnish with thin slice of lemon.

Cakes and Biscuits

Spice Bread

SERVES 12

300mL (1¼ cups) boiling water
180g (¾ cup) honey
200g (1 cup) sugar
60mL (¼ cup) rum
1 teaspoon cinnamon
1 teaspoon ginger (optional)
480g (4 cups) self-raising white flour, sifted
2 teaspoons bicarbonate of soda
2 tablespoons candied peel, chopped
½ teaspoon orange rind, finely grated

Stir together the water, honey, sugar, rum, cinnamon and ginger. Mix well then stir in the flour and bicarbonate of soda. Mix well to make a smooth batter, then add peel and rind. Place in a greased loaf tin and bake in a hot oven (220°C) for about 10 minutes. Reduce the heat to moderate (180°C) and bake for further 1 hour or until when tested a skewer comes out clean.

Danish Crescents

SERVES 10

250g (1 cup) salt-free polyunsaturated margarine
400g (2⅔ cups) plain white flour
50g (2½ tablespoons) castor sugar
70g (3½ tablespoons) strawberry jam
½ egg, beaten lightly

Rub margarine into flour. Add sugar and knead lightly. Roll out and cut into 10 triangles (12cm base). Spread jam along base. Roll up loosely from base to point. Shape into crescents. Glaze with beaten egg. Bake on a greased biscuit tray in a hot oven (220°C) for 20 to 25 minutes or until light brown.

Mandarin Cake

SERVES 12

250g (1 cup) salt-free polyunsaturated margarine
180g (¾ cup) castor sugar
3 × 55g eggs, lightly beaten
225g (1½ cups) self-raising white flour, sieved
20mL (1 tablespoon) hot water

Topping

250mL (1 cup) cream
10g (2 teaspoons) castor sugar
300g (1 can) mandarin segments, well drained

Grease a 20cm diameter cake tin. Cream the margarine and sugar until pale and fluffy. Add eggs, one at a time, and beat well. Fold in the sieved flour. Add a little water until the cake is a soft consistency. Pour the batter into the cake tin and bake in a moderate oven (180°C) for approximately 50 minutes or until it comes away from the sides of the tin. Turn out and cool on a wire rack.

Whip the cream and sugar until it stands in firm peaks. Spread over the top of the cake. Decorate with the mandarin segments.

Chewy Noels

SERVES 12

2 × 55g eggs
1 teaspoon vanilla essence
170g (1 cup) brown sugar
60g (½ cup) self-raising white flour
40g (2 tablespoons) salt-free polyunsaturated margarine
Icing sugar

Beat eggs and vanilla together lightly. Combine the brown sugar and flour. Add this to the egg and vanilla mixture. Mix well. Melt the margarine and pour into base of a bar pan (8 × 26cm). Pour in the mixture and bake in a moderate oven (180°C) till firm to touch, approximately 25 minutes. Turn out to cool with the buttered side up. Dust lightly with the icing sugar. Cut into squares and serve.

Apple Shortcakes

SERVES 12

250g (2 cups) self-raising white flour
125g (½ cup) salt-free polyunsaturated margarine
30g (2 tablespoons) castor sugar
1 × 55g egg
80mL (⅓ cup) milk
Milk for brushing
125mL (½ cup) cream, whipped
250g (1 cup) stewed or canned apple, well drained
15g (1 tablespoon) icing sugar

Sift flour and rub in the margarine. Beat the egg, milk and sugar and then slowly mix into the flour and the margarine. Mix till a soft dough forms. Turn out onto a floured board and knead the dough, then roll out until 1cm thick. Cut into twelve rounds with biscuit cutter or small scone cutter. Place in a greased baking tray and brush tops with milk. Bake in a moderately hot oven (180°C) for 15 minutes. Cool on a wire rack. Once they are cool enough to handle, split each shortcake in half. Use your hands to do this, not a knife.

When completely cool, sandwich the shortcakes together with the cream and apple. Dust the tops with icing sugar before serving.

Ginger Slice

SERVES 12

125g (½ cup) salt-free polyunsaturated margarine
120g (⅔ cup) castor sugar
210g (1⅓ cups) plain white flour
1 teaspoon baking powder
1 teaspoon ground ginger

Icing

30g (1½ tablespoons) salt-free polyunsaturated margarine
60g (⅓ cup) icing sugar
15g (2 teaspoons) golden syrup
1 teaspoon ground ginger

Cream margarine and sugar into a mixing bowl. Add sifted dry ingredients. Mix well and press into a greased 20 × 20cm baking tin. Bake in a moderate oven (180°C) for 20 to 25 minutes.

Put margarine, icing sugar, golden syrup and ginger in a saucepan. Heat over a low heat until melted, then pour over slice whilst still warm. Allow to cool slightly. Cut into slices while still warm.

Cream Puffs

MAKES 12

300mL (1¼ cups) water
85g (⅓ cup) salt-free polyunsaturated margarine
150g (1 cup) plain white flour
4 × 55g eggs
600mL (2½ cups) cream
60g (⅓ cup) icing sugar

Mix the water and margarine in a saucepan and melt over medium heat. Sieve the flour onto a piece of greaseproof paper. When the water is boiling and margarine dissolved, quickly pour the flour into the saucepan, stirring rapidly with a wooden spoon. Continue stirring until the mixture forms a smooth ball and leaves the sides of the saucepan. Remove from heat. Allow to cool for 2 minutes. Beat eggs slightly and add to the mixture, approximately one at a time, and beat well until thoroughly absorbed. Continue to beat in the eggs until a satin-like shine develops.

Preheat the oven to 220°C. Lightly grease a baking tray. Place a 1cm plain piping tube into a forcing bag. Put the choux pastry into the bag and pipe small pieces (about the size of a large walnut) onto the tray at least 8cm apart. Sprinkle the puffs and tray liberally with water. Cover the puffs with an inverted roasting pan to keep the steam in. Bake for 20 to 25 minutes, then reduce the temperature to moderate (180°C) and bake for a further 10 minutes. The puffs should be crisp, and of light, even colour. Remove from baking tray to a wire cooling rack. When cool, cut the puffs open across the centre. Discard 'sticky' centre.

Whip the cream. Pipe into the cream puffs and sprinkle liberally with icing sugar.

CHAPTER

4

DIET AND RECIPES FOR THE PERSON ON CONTINUOUS AMBULATORY PERITONEAL DIALYSIS (CAPD)

Maintaining and increased protein intake	94
Fluctuations of body weight	95
Elevated blood fats	97
Elevated blood sugars	97
Special supplements	98
Eating out	98
Takeaway and restaurant food guide for the weight-conscious CAPD patient	99
High-protein recipes	
Soups and starters	105
Omelettes	111
Stuffed vegetables	113
Savoury melts	115
Savoury jaffles	117
Desserts	119
Beverages	125

Continuous ambulatory peritoneal dialysis (CAPD) removes waste products and fluid from the body on a day-to-day basis. One of the major advantages of this is that waste and fluids are less likely to build up to high levels as happens with haemodialysis. Thus CAPD patients can enjoy a relatively free diet. A 'free diet' does not mean that food intake can be neglected.

People on CAPD have increased needs for protein and certain vitamins (particularly vitamins B and C). The reason for this is that these nutrients are continually being lost from the body into the dialysis fluid. A well-balanced diet that is adequate in protein is needed to maintain good nutrition. This reduces the risk of developing infections or becoming ill.

Dietary modification may be required for CAPD patients, especially for those who experience fluctuations in body weight and/or increased levels of fat or sugar in the blood.

The dietary management of the most common diet-related problems experienced by people on CAPD is discussed below.

MAINTAINING AN INCREASED PROTEIN INTAKE

Include adequate amounts of protein-rich foods.

Your doctor or dietitian will advise you on the amounts of the protein-rich foods you need to consume.

Protein-rich Foods

Meat
Poultry
Milk and milk products
Cheese
Seafood
Legumes (e.g., soya, broad and kidney beans, lentils, etc.)
Eggs
Nuts

Maintaining an adequate protein intake may be difficult for those with small appetites or during episodes of peritonitis where protein requirements are increased. In these cases the following suggestions may help.

Choose light alternatives to the typical 'meat' meal.

Omelette or egg dishes
Pasta with meat, seafood or cheese sauce

The Person on CAPD

> Hearty soups thickened with milk and/or cheese
> Vegetables with cheese sauce
> Sandwiches with protein-rich fillings, e.g., meat, poultry, salmon or tuna, egg, baked beans or cheese
> Meals including liberal amounts of legumes or nuts

Choose high-protein snacks between meals.

> Biscuits and cheese   Yoghurt
> Nuts   Ice cream
> Custard   Milk-based desserts

Include these spreads with bread or crackers.

> Peanut butter   Hummus (chick pea dip)
> Cheese spread   Taramasalata (fishroe dip)
> Pate   Tazatziki (yoghurt dip)
> Cottage or Ricotta cheese

Choose high-protein beverages to drink.

> Milk-based hearty soups   Milk coffee
> Milkshakes or thickshakes   Hot chocolate
> Egg flips   Commercially made
> Flavoured milk   supplement drinks

Recipes and further ideas can be found in the recipe section.

FLUCTUATIONS OF BODY WEIGHT

Fluid retention

Most people experience fluctuations of body weight on peritoneal dialysis. Rapid changes are usually the result of gains or losses of fluid rather than changes of body fat or tissue. Fluid retention that results in elevation of weight, blood pressure and swelling (usually in feet, hands or face) may necessitate restriction of daily fluid intake. Avoiding table salt as well as highly salted snack and processed foods will also help if fluid retention is a problem.

Weight gain

The dialysate fluid used by people on CAPD is actually a sugar solution. Gradual gains in body fat may occur as a result of sugars absorbed into the bloodstream from the dialysis fluid. Gains of body fat may also be related to an excessive energy (kilojoule/ calorie) intake and to a decrease in physical activity.

Reduction of body fat can be achieved by increased physical activity and a restriction of energy intake. This should not, however, jeopardize the protein content or nutritional balance of the diet. The guidelines below for reducing fat, sugar and alcohol intake will assist with weight (fat) loss, whilst maintaining the nutritional quality of the diet.

Reducing Fat Intake

Use fat-reduced dairy foods
Grill or steam foods instead of frying
Use lean meats trimmed of visible fat
Remove skin from poultry
Use only a scrape of polyunsaturated margarine or butter on bread.

Reducing Sugar Intake

Avoid added sugar
Avoid confectionary and rich desserts
Avoid sweetened breakfast cereals
Avoid drinks with added sugar such as soft drinks and cordials
Limit alcohol consumption

Weight Loss

Decreased appetite due to a feeling of fullness experienced when dialysis fluid is in the abdomen can, on the contrary, result in weight loss. Maintaining an adequate intake of high-protein food will help to prevent this.

If weight loss is a problem, try supplementing the diet with high-protein drinks, e.g., milkshakes and egg flips; and eating high-protein snacks between meals, e.g., nuts, cheese, yoghurt.

Timing of meals to occur when dialysis fluid is draining out is often helpful.

ELEVATED BLOOD FATS

Cholesterol and triglycerides are two different types of fat, the levels of which may be elevated in the blood of persons on CAPD. Elevated levels of these fats have been associated with an increased risk of heart and vascular disease.

People who have elevated blood cholesterol should try to reduce it by:

1. Achieving or maintaining an ideal body weight.
2. Reducing intake of fat, particularly saturated (animal) fats and cholesterol (see also hints on reducing fat intake, page 96).
3. Using polyunsaturated or monounsaturated fats (e.g., polyunsaturated oil, margarine or olive oil) instead of butter and solid frying oils (see also hints on reducing fat intake, page 96).

Those with elevated triglyceride levels should also try to reduce their intake of refined sugars and alcohol.

ELEVATED BLOOD SUGARS

Dialysate fluids contain sugar and can elevate blood sugar levels in some people. Reduction of the simple sugars consumed in the diet can help to reduce blood sugar levels (see hints on reducing sugar intake, page 96).

SPECIAL SUPPLEMENTS

Commercially available high-protein drinks or vitamin/mineral supplements may be useful for patients on CAPD. The use of these should be at the recommendation of your doctor or dietitian.

EATING OUT

Some people may be hesitant to eat out whilst they are on CAPD. This may be because they have a poor appetite or because they are concerned about weight gain or fluid balance.

There is no reason why you should not enjoy eating out occasionally whilst on CAPD. The following suggestions may help.

Tips for Small Appetites

1. You may find it easier to choose two entrees rather than an entree and a main course.
2. Going to ethnic restaurants where dishes are often shared allows you to choose a variety of foods and eat to your appetite.
3. Try to avoid drinking fluids with meals—these can cause you to feel full and make it difficult for you to finish your meal.
4. Take time over the meal.

Tips for the Overweight

1. Select meals that have a lower fat and sugar content.
2. Try to have one or two rather than three courses.
3. Try to avoid cream sauces, battered or fried foods, rich cakes and puddings or cheese platters.

Further tips can be found in the takeaway and restaurant food guide.

Tips for Decreasing Fluid Intake

1. Beware of having your glass topped up—this makes it difficult to estimate how much you are drinking.
2. Try to avoid choosing very salty foods as these will increase your thirst.

3. Reduce your fluid intake at other times of the day, if you wish to drink more when you have a special meal out.
4. Large amounts of ice in drinks need to be counted as extra fluid.
5. Further suggestions can be found under Helpful Hints For Fluid Control (page 58).

TAKEAWAY AND RESTAURANT FOOD GUIDE FOR THE WEIGHT-CONSCIOUS CAPD PATIENT

This guide to takeaway and restaurant foods should be helpful to those who are watching their weight. Some of the more appropriate choices may contain more kilojoules (calories) and salt than would be recommended in your daily meal plan. However, this should not be a problem if you eat out only occasionally. If you are on a fluid restriction you need to limit your intake of soups, drinks, and desserts containing milk or fruit.

Asian Cuisine

Best Choice

Soups	Steamed fish
Steamed dim sims	Braised or steamed vegetables
Chop suey, chow mein	Steamed rice
Omelettes	Lychees
Braises, satay	Plain ice cream

Suitable Very Occasionally

Fried Dim Sims	Sweet and sour dishes
Spring rolls	Prawn Cutlets
Gow Gee	Fried rice
Soya sauce	Fried ice cream

Cafe, Cafeteria, Foodstand

Best Choice

Consomme	Plain scone
Sandwich or bread roll	Fresh fruit

Toasted sandwich
Salad
Cheese stick
Hamburger with salad
Hot dog
BBQ chicken (no skin)
Raisin bread, fruit bun

Low-fat yoghurt
Plain ice cream
Plain or skim milk
Fruit juice (no added sugar)
Diet drinks
Coffee or tea

Suitable Very Occasionally

Pie or pastie
Sausage roll
Chiko roll
Fried fish
Fish cocktails
Potato scallops

French fries
Confectionary
Rich cakes
Potato, corn chips
Soft drinks
Cream in coffee

French Cuisine

Best Choice

Consomme
Frogs' legs
Snails
Savoury crepe
Grilled lean meat
Grilled or steamed fish

Vegetables or salad
Plain bread or bread rolls
Fresh fruit
Ice cream
Crepes with fresh fruit
Sauces

Suitable Very Occasionally

Vol au vents
Souffles
Cream sauces
French fries

Garlic or herb bread
Profiteroles
Rich cakes or pastry

Greek and Lebanese Cuisine

Best Choice

Soup
Dolmades

Grilled octopus or calamari
Grilled lean meat

Taramasalata ⎫
Hommus and ⎬ small amount
tahini ⎭
Yoghurt dip
Souvlaki
Tabouli
Doner Kebab

Grilled chicken (no skin)
Grilled or steamed fish
Stuffed vegetables
Small amount fetta cheese
Bread or bread rolls
Lebanese or Pita bread
Fresh fruit

Suitable Very Occasionally

Cheese and spinach triangles
Felafel
Moussaka
Fried calamari
Fried potato

Garlic bread
Turkish delight
Baklawa
Rich cakes

Italian Cuisine

Best Choice

Minestrone
Pasta with meat or tomato sauce
Veal with tomato sauce
Grilled fish or chicken
Pizza (small serve)

Salad
Bread roll
Fresh fruit
Gelato
Zabaglioni

Suitable Very Occasionally

Salami
Mortadella
Italian sausage
Pasta with cream sauce
Pizza with extra topping

Fried meats or chicken
Fried seafood or calamari
Profiteroles
Rich cakes or tortes

Indian Cuisine

Best Choice

Tomato Sambal
Cucumber Raita

Mixed vegetable curry
Chapatis

Chutneys or Dahl
Beef, lamb, chicken or
   seafood curry
Tandoori chicken

Steamed rice
Fresh fruit
Custards

Suitable Very Occasionally

Bhayas (fried vegetables)
Roti

Papadams
Rich cakes

International Cuisine

Best Choice

Consomme
Grilled or BBQ meat
Lean roast meat or chicken
   (no skin)
Boiled vegetables or salad

Fresh or canned fruit
Ice cream
Yoghurt
Very *small* cheese platter

Suitable Very Occasionally

Fried meat or schnitzel
Fried seafood
Chicken Maryland
Cream or rich butter sauces
Garlic or herb bread

Rich cakes or Torte
Pastry
Pavlova
Cheesecake

Japanese Cuisine

Best Choice

Tofu
Sushi or sashimi

Sukiyaki
Steamboat

Suitable Very Occasionally

Miso

Tempura

Seafood

Best Choice

Oysters natural
Seafood or prawn cocktail
Seafood crepe (no sauce)
Grilled, poached or BBQ fish
Steamed seafood platter
Seafood salad

Steamed vegetables or salad
Bread or bread roll
Fresh fruit
Sorbet
Ice cream

Suitable Very Occasionally

Fried calamari
Prawn cutlets
Oysters mornay
Oyster kilpatrick
Seafood with cream sauce

Fritto misto
Crumbed or battered fish
Garlic or herb bread
Rich cakes or desserts

Mexican Cuisine

Best Choice

Tacos
Buritos
Grilled meat, chicken or
   seafood

Topo salad

Suitable Very Occasionally

Guacamole
Sour cream

Nachos
Frijoles (fried beans)

Vegetarian Cuisine

Best Choice

Clear soup
Steamed vegetables or salad

Fruit salad
Yoghurt

Rice or pasta   Ice cream
Fresh fruit

Suitable Very Occasionally

Fried vegetables   Rich cakes
Pastry   Desserts

Soups and Starters

Red Salmon Dip

SERVES 8

220g (1 can) low-salt red salmon, drained
100g (½ small carton) low-fat natural yoghurt
3–4 spring onions, chopped
Pinch mixed herbs
Freshly ground black pepper to taste

Combine all ingredients. Serve as a dip with vegetables or a spread for bread.

For a smoother dip place all ingredients in blender or food processor and process briefly.

Cheese Fondue

SERVES 2–4

1 clove garlic
200g (2 cups) grated cheese
20g (2 tablespoons) plain white flour
Large pinch ground nutmeg
Large pinch pepper
180mL (¾ cup) low-fat milk
French bread

Cut the clove of garlic in half and rub the inside of the fondue pot very well with the cut garlic. Discard the garlic. Combine cheese, flour, nutmeg and pepper in a plastic bag and shake well to mix thoroughly. Heat the milk in the fondue pot till just boiling. Maintain over heat, add the mix from the plastic bag and whisk well with a fork until the cheese dissolves and the mix is bubbling. Place the pot over a fondue candle. Serve with chunks of crusty French bread.

Fish Stock

SERVES 8

- 1 kg mixed fish bones (include some flesh, heads and trimmings; and a few uncooked prawns and calamari rings)
- 2 cleaned and trimmed mussels
- 1 large white onion, thinly sliced
- 1 stalk celery with leaves, sliced
- 1 cup dry white wine
- 6 black peppercorns
- 1 sprig fresh thyme
- 2 sprigs fresh parsley
- 8 cups water
- Juice 1 lemon

Place all ingredients in a large saucepan and bring to the boil. Reduce heat, cover and simmer for 20 minutes. Skim the surface and strain through a fine sieve. Store in refrigerator and use as required.

Makes approximately 8 cups.

Chicken or Beef Stock

SERVES 8

- 1 kg skinned chicken pieces and bones or beef, trimmed of all visible fat
- 1 large white onion, sliced
- 1 carrot, sliced
- 1 stalk celery with leaves, chopped
- 1 bay leaf
- 3 sprigs fresh parsley, chopped
- 4 peppercorns
- 9 cups water

Place all ingredients in a large saucepan and bring to the boil. Reduce heat, cover and simmer for 1½ hours. Strain the stock through a fine sieve and allow to cool. Refrigerate overnight and in the morning skim off the surface fat.

Makes approximately 8 cups.

Lentil Soup

SERVES 4

60g (1 small) carrot, diced
120g (1 medium) onion, sliced
60g (1 small) turnip, diced
1L (4 cups) chicken, beef or vegetable stock
½ teaspoon dried thyme
½ teaspoon pepper
200g (1 cup) uncooked lentils, red or green
300mL (1¼ cups) low-fat milk
Chopped parsley to garnish

Saute carrot, onion and turnip in a small amount of stock. When tender add remaining ingredients, except for the milk. Cook until lentils are tender. Press through a sieve or put into the blender. Reheat, thin down with milk, garnish with parsley and serve.

Almond Soup

SERVES 4–6

120g (1) leek
160g (4 sticks) celery
125g (2 cups) ground blanched almonds
1L (4 cups) low-fat milk
Cayenne pepper
30g (¼ cup) toasted flaked almonds
Nutmeg as desired

Finely chop the leek and celery. Place ground almonds, milk, leek and celery in a saucepan and simmer over low heat until vegetables are tender. Puree in blender. Season with cayenne pepper. The soup may be served hot or well chilled. Sprinkle with toasted almonds and nutmeg to serve.

Pea Soup

SERVES 6

280g (2 ⅔ cups) green split peas
120g (1 medium) onion, chopped
60g (1 small) carrot, chopped
125g lean bacon, chopped
1½L (6 cups) water
Pepper to taste
2 tablespoons chopped mint to garnish

Wash peas well. Place in a saucepan with onion, carrot, bacon and water. Bring slowly to the boil. Skim well. Cover pan and cook until peas are tender, approximately 2 hours. Sieve or blend soup then return to heat. Season with pepper. Garnish with chopped mint before serving.

Combination Seafood Soup

SERVES 6–8

250g green prawns
2L (8 cups) water
500g fish fillets
1 bayleaf
90g (4½ tablespoons) polyunsaturated margarine
1 teaspoon curry powder
60g (½ cup) plain white flour
120g (⅓ cup) tomato paste
Few drops tabasco sauce
180g (2 medium) potatoes, peeled and diced
160g (2 medium) carrots, diced
Pepper to taste
250g scallops
250g mussels
170g (⅔ cup) low-fat natural yoghurt
2 tablespoons parsley, chopped

Shell and clean prawns, reserving prawn shells. Put water, fish fillets, prawn shells and bayleaf into a large pan, bring to boil, reduce heat, and simmer, covered, for 10 minutes. Strain, reserve stock and fish fillets. Heat margarine in a large pan, add curry powder and flour, stirring until combined. Remove pan from heat. Add reserved stock and stir until combined. Return pan to heat, add tomato paste, tabasco sauce, potatoes, and carrots, and stir until mixture boils. Reduce heat and simmer gently, covered, for 30 minutes. Season with pepper.

Cut prawns into pieces, clean scallops and cut in half, clean mussels and flake reserved fish fillets. Add to the soup. Simmer a further 5 minutes, uncovered, or until mussel shells open. Add yoghurt and parsley and stir until combined.

Tasty Meat and Vegetable Soup

SERVES 8

120g (1 medium) onion, finely chopped
1 clove garlic, chopped
2L (8 cups) fresh beef stock (see page 106)
500g lean minced steak
½ teaspoon black pepper
1 teaspoon dried oregano
½ teaspoon dried basil
180g (3 small) zucchini, thinly sliced
120g (¾ cup) shelled peas (or frozen peas)
135g (1 medium) tomato, peeled and coarsley chopped
60g (½ cup) parmesan cheese, grated

In a large saucepan saute onion and garlic in a small amount of beef stock over moderate heat. Add meat and cook, stirring occasionally, until meat is broken up and brown. Pour in the stock and add pepper, herbs, zucchini and peas. Bring to the boil. Reduce heat to low and simmer for 15 minutes. Add tomato and simmer for a further 5 minutes. Sprinkle with cheese just before serving.

Tip

To reduce the fat content, chill soup after tomatoes have simmered then skim any fat from the surface. Reheat and sprinkle with cheese just before serving.

Cream of Chicken and Corn Soup

SERVES 6–8

450g can corn kernels (no added salt)
1½L (6 cups) fresh chicken stock (see page 106)
¾ teaspoon grated ginger
4 shallots, chopped
1 cup diced cooked chicken (without skin)
Pepper to taste
4 tablespoons cornflour
300mL (1¼ cups) low-fat milk
2 egg whites
Parsley to garnish

Combine corn, stock, ginger, shallots, chicken and pepper in a large saucepan and bring to the boil. Mix cornflour with a little water to form a paste, then add to the soup. Stir until soup boils and thickens. Reduce heat and simmer for 1 to 2 minutes. Add milk, do not boil. Slowly add egg whites beaten with a little water, stirring well. Serve hot garnished with parsley.

Savoury Omelettes

Basic Omelette

SERVES 1

2 × 60 eggs
White pepper
2 teaspoons salt-free polyunsaturated margarine

Beat eggs and pepper vigorously with fork until mixture is frothy. Heat margarine over a moderate heat until foaming (if using a non-stick frying pan, warm pan without margarine). Pour egg mix into pan and move in a circular motion with a fork until mixture begins to thicken. Stop stirring, leave over heat for another 30 seconds, then remove from heat. Free bottom and edges of omelette from pan by tapping the bottom of the pan on the edge of the stove and/or use a fork or spatula. Toss omelette over on to the other side and return to heat for another 10 seconds. Slide omelette onto a plate and serve immediately.

Omelette Variations

Combine the ingredients for each of the variations and add to the omelette while in the pan, before turning it over. All recipes serve 1.

Chicken, Corn and Capsicum

    30g (¼ cup) cooked chicken, without skin, finely diced
    1 dessertspoon corn kernels (no added salt)
    1 dessertspoon capsicum, finely chopped

Curried Tuna and Celery

    50g (½ small tin) tuna (no added salt), drained
    1 teaspoon curry powder
    ½ stick celery, finely chopped

Cheese, Mushroom and Tomato

>40g (½ cup) grated cheese (preferably reduced fat, reduced salt variety)
>1 large mushroom, diced
>½ small tomato, diced

Salmon and Spring Onion

>60g (½ small tin) salmon (no added salt), drained
>1–2 spring onions, diced

Ham, Asparagus and Mustard

>30g (1 slice) lean ham, diced (reduced fat and salt variety preferable)
>1 teaspoon dry mustard
>2 spears asparagus, chopped

Stuffed Vegetables

If using potatoes, wash, scrub and bake them in their jackets in oven until tender when pierced with a skewer. Slice top off potatoes and scoop out flesh, but leave a firm casing to be filled.

If using tomatoes, slice the top off and scoop out the flesh, leaving a firm casing. If using capsicums, slice the top off then core and deseed case.

Mash potato or tomato flesh with suggested fillings. If filling is a little dry add 1 or 2 tablespoons skim milk. Fill the potato, tomato or capsicum cases, place in a hot oven (220°C) and bake for 10 to 15 minutes or until tops are golden brown.

Each of the suggested fillings fills one large potato, capsicum or tomato.

Filling Suggestions

ALL RECIPES SERVE ONE

Tuna Ricotta Filling

    1 tablespoon tuna (no added salt)
    1 tablespoon ricotta cheese
    2 teaspoons chopped chives
    1 egg white
    Black pepper to taste

Nutty Ricotta Filling

    1 tablespoon crunchy peanut butter
    1 tablespoon ricotta cheese
    ½ stick celery, chopped
    1 egg white

Curried Salmon Filling

> 1 tablespoon salmon (no added salt), drained
> 1 tablespoon low-fat cottage cheese
> ¼ teaspoon curry power
> ¼ green apple, diced
> 1 egg white

Chilli Cheese Filling

> ½ small tomato, chopped
> ¼ cup grated cheese (reduced salt and fat varieties are preferable)
> ¼ teaspoon chilli power
> 1 egg white

Pizziola

> ¼ cup grated mozarella cheese
> ½ small tomato, diced
> 1 slice (30g) ham, diced (reduced fat and salt variety preferable)
> 1 tablespoon diced capsicum
> 1 egg white

Sprinkle with 1 teaspoon Parmesan cheese before reheating.

Creamy Chicken with Dill Filling

> ¼ cup diced cooked and skinned chicken
> 1 tablespoon ricotta cheese
> ¼ teaspoon Dijon mustard
> 1 egg white
> 1 teaspoon fresh chopped dill

Savoury Melts

Place the following on toasted bread, muffins, crumpets or bread rolls and grill.

Baked Bean Melt

¼ cup baked beans
1 slice (30g) cheese (reduced fat and salt variety preferable)

Grill until cheese melts.

Paprika Chicken Melt

1 tablespoon chopped cooked and skinned chicken
1 tablespoon of cottage cheese
Pinch paprika
1 slice (30g) cheese (reduced fat and salt variety preferable)

Grill till golden brown.

Pizza Melt

1 slice ham, diced
¼ cup grated Mozarella cheese
½ small tomato, diced
½ teaspoon Parmesan cheese

Combine and grill until cheese melts and is golden brown. Diced capsicum, onion and pineapple may be added.

Salmon and Avocado Melt

1 tablespoon mashed avocado
1 tablespoon salmon (no added salt)
Black pepper to taste
1 slice (30g) cheese

Grill until golden brown.

Tuna and Gherkin Melt

1 tablespoon tuna
3 chopped gherkins
1 slice (30g) cheese

Grill until golden brown.

Savoury Jaffles

Combine the ingredients of each of the following variations. Place inside 2 slices of bread with the outside spread with margarine. Cook in a jaffle iron or a toasted sandwich maker.

Cheese and Chutney

¼ cup low-fat cottage or ricotta cheese
2 heaped teaspoons chutney

Ham, Cheese and Pineapple

¼ cup low-fat cottage cheese
1 slice ham
1 slice pineapple

Cheese and Raisin

¼ cup low-fat cottage cheese
½ small carrot, grated
1 tablespoon raisins

Egg

1 × 60g egg
Black pepper

Baked Beans and Cheese

110g (1 small can) baked beans
1 slice cheese (preferably reduced fat and reduced salt)

Cheese and Walnuts

¼ cup low-fat cottage or ricotta cheese
1 tablespoon walnuts

Cheese, Tomato and Celery

½ stick celery, chopped
Sliced tomato
1 slice hard cheese (preferably reduced fat and salt)

Tuna and Spring Onion

110g (1 small can) no added salt tuna (drained)
1–2 spring onions, chopped
Black pepper

Salmon and Cucumber

¼ cup no added salt salmon (drained)
2–3 slices cucumber

Desserts

High-Protein Custard

SERVES 4

1 tablespoon custard powder
600mL (2⅓ cups) low-fat milk
80g (½ cup) skim-milk powder
Sugar or artificial sweetener to taste

Mix custard powder with a little milk until a smooth paste forms. Add the milk powder to the rest of the milk and heat gently until it begins to boil. Add the custard powder mix and stir until thickened. Sweeten with sugar or artificial sweetener.

Baked Rice Custard

SERVES 4

250mL (1 cup) water
30g (2 tablespoons) uncooked short-grain rice
3 × 60g eggs
70g (⅓ cup) sugar, or liquid artificial sweetener to taste
1 teaspoon vanilla
40g (¼ cup) sultanas
625mL (2½ cups) low-fat milk
Nutmeg or cinnamon

Place water in a saucepan and, when rapidly boiling, add rice and boil for 10 minutes. Drain well. Whisk eggs, sugar and vanilla together, add rice and sultanas, gradually whisk in milk. Pour into a shallow oven-proof dish and sprinkle with cinnamon or nutmeg. Stand in a baking dish with enough water to come half way up the sides of the dish. Bake in a moderate oven (180°C) for 45 to 60 minutes or until set and golden brown.

Variations

BANANA RICE PUDDING
    200g (2 medium) bananas, thinly sliced
    40mL (2 tablespoons) lemon juice
    20g (1 tablespoon) brown sugar
    Extra nutmeg

APPLE RICE PUDDING
    150g (1 medium) apple, thinly sliced
    40mL (2 tablespoons) lemon juice
    20g (1 tablespoon) brown sugar
    Extra cinnamon

Toss bananas or apple in lemon juice 5 minutes before custard has finished cooking (but should be firm to touch). Place fruit on top and sprinkle with sugar and spice.

Return to oven and complete cooking, approximately 5 minutes.

Bread and Butter Custard

SERVES 4

    4 slices bread
    Salt-free polyunsaturated margarine
    2 tablespoons sultanas
    500mL (2 cups) low-fat milk
    4 × 60g eggs
    50g (¼ cup) sugar or liquid artificial sweetener to taste
    1 teaspoon vanilla
    Nutmeg or cinnamon

Trim crusts from bread and spread thinly with margarine. Cut each slice into 4 triangles. Sprinkle sultanas into ovenproof dish. Place bread on top, buttered side up. Lightly beat milk, eggs, sugar or sweetener and vanilla. Pour over the bread. Let stand for about 10 minutes. Sprinkle the top with nutmeg or cinnamon. Bake in a moderate oven (180°C) for 40 minutes or until the custard is set and the top is golden brown.

Fruit Fool

SERVES 4

300mL (1¼ cups) fruit puree
A little sugar or artificial sweetener to taste
125mL (½ cup) skim evaporated milk
Spices to taste

Sweeten the fruit puree to taste. Whip the evaporated milk and fold into fruit puree. Pour into individual glasses and chill. Sprinkle with spice before serving.

Chocolate Blancmange

SERVES 4

40g (⅓ cup) cornflour
500mL (2 cups) low-fat milk
1 teaspoon vanilla essence
40mL 2 tablespoons chocolate syrup
A little grated chocolate for serving

Blend cornflour in a bowl with ½ cup of milk. Heat the remaining milk in the pan. When nearly boiling quickly stir in cornflour mixture and continue to stir over heat until mixture boils and thickens; stir over heat for a further 1 minute. Remove from heat and add vanilla essence and chocolate syrup. Pour mixture into 4 individual serving dishes that have been rinsed out with cold water (do not dry). Refrigerate until firm.

Sprinkle with grated chocolate to serve.

Mocha Mousse

SERVES 4

1 tablespoon gelatine
65mL (¼ cup) hot water
2 teaspoons instant coffee
500g low-fat banana yoghurt
40mL (2 tablespoons) coffee liqueur
80mL (⅓ cup) skim evaporated milk, chilled
Banana slices to decorate
Juice of 1 lemon
Cinnamon to decorate

Sprinkle gelatine over hot water and stir until dissolved to a clear liquid. Stir in coffee and yoghurt until smooth. Add the liqueur.

Whip chilled evaporated milk with the electric beater until doubled in volume. Fold into yoghurt mixture. Pour into 4 individual serving dishes and chill to set. Decorate with banana slices dipped in lemon juice and sprinkle with cinnamon.

Fruit Yoghurt Ice Cream

SERVES 4

2½ teaspoons gelatine
125mL (½ cup) hot water
200g (1 small carton) low-fat natural yoghurt
80g (½ cup) skim milk powder
50g (½ cup) castor sugar
1 teaspoon vanilla essence
250g fresh or unsweetened canned fruit

Sprinkle gelatine over hot water and dissolve; cool 5 minutes. Place gelatine mix into a bowl and stir in yoghurt, milk powder, sugar and vanilla until smooth. Pour mixture into a lamington tin, cover with foil. Freeze for approximately 45 minutes or until almost set. Remove from freezer and place the mixture in a bowl. Mix with an electric mixer on high speed until it has doubled in bulk. Puree fruit of your choice (if there are seeds, sieve to remove them).

Combine the fruit with the ice cream and pour into loaf pan. Cover with foil and freeze several hours or until firm.

Stuffed Peaches

SERVES 1

200g (1 large) fresh peach
2 teaspoons smooth ricotta cheese
2 teaspoons low-fat natural yoghurt
1 teaspoon lemon juice
Liquid sweetener to taste
Chopped walnuts for garnish

Peel and halve peach and remove the stone. Place the 2 halves on a serving plate. Combine remaining ingredients and sweeten if needed. Place into the cavity of each peach half. Grill or bake for 5 to 10 minutes. Garnish with chopped walnuts.

Pumpkin Cheesecake

SERVES 12

125g WeetBix or Vita Brits
60g (3 tablespoons) polyunsaturated margarine, melted
¼ teaspoon allspice
500g pumpkin
2 × 60g eggs
¼ cup honey (or the equivalent in liquid sweetener)
1 teaspoon nutmeg
750g ricotta cheese
¼ teaspoon extra nutmeg

Crush biscuits in a food processor or with a rolling pin. Add margarine, allspice and mix well. Press evenly onto base and sides of a 20cm spring-form tin.

Remove seeds from pumpkin (but do not peel), cut into pieces and cook in boiling water for 15 minutes until tender. Drain well and, when cool, trim away skin. Blend pumpkin in food processor or mash with potato masher. Add remaining ingredients, except extra nutmeg, and combine well either in food processor or with a rotary beater.

Spoon filling into biscuit case, smooth top and sprinkle with extra nutmeg. Bake in a moderate oven (180°C) until firm.

Allow to cool then refrigerate for several hours before serving.

Tropical Fruit Slice

SERVES 8

60g (3) crushed WeetBix or Vita Brits
60g (3 tablespoons) polyunsaturated margarine
250mL (1 cup) low-fat fruit salad yoghurt
250g low-fat ricotta or cottage cheese
40g (2 tablespoons) honey
½ teaspoon vanilla essence
1 teaspoon orange rind
1 tablespoon gelatine
40mL (2 tablespoons) hot water
Passionfruit to garnish

Combine WeetBix or Vita Brits with margarine and press evenly onto base of a foil-lined 20cm loaf tin.

Beat the yoghurt, cheese, honey, vanilla and grated orange rind until smooth and creamy. Sprinkle gelatine over hot water and stir until dissolved. Let cool slightly. Fold through yoghurt mixture and pour over base. Top with passionfruit if desired.

Refrigerate until firm. Cut into slices and serve.

Beverages

Basic Milkshake

SERVES 1

250mL (1 cup) low-fat milk
80g (½ cup) skim-milk powder
60g (1 scoop) ice cream
Flavouring or topping to taste, low joule varieties are available

Blend all ingredients and serve.

Fruit Shake

As for milkshake but add your favourite fruit, e.g. banana, pineapple or rockmelon.

Orange Egg Nog

SERVES 1

1 × 60g egg
125mL (½ cup) unsweetened orange juice
125mL (½ cup) skim evaporated milk
20mL (1 tablespoon) brandy

Blend all ingredients together and serve.

Yoghurt Shake

SERVES 1

100g (½ small) carton natural low-fat yoghurt
125mL (½ cup) unsweetened fruit juice
125mL (½ cup) pureed fresh or unsweetened fruit

Blend all ingredients together and serve.

Iced Coffee

SERVES 1

1 teaspoon instant coffee
250mL (1 cup) low-fat milk
1 tablespoon skim milk powder
1 scoop ice cream
Nutmeg to garnish

Dissolve instant coffee in some warm water. Add skim milk powder to low-fat milk then mix with coffee. Top with ice cream and sprinkle with nutmeg.

Cafe Au Lait

SERVES 1

1 teaspoon instant coffee
200mL low-fat milk

Dissolve instant coffee in some warm water. Heat milk until warm, mix in coffee and serve.

Liqueur Coffee

To cafe au lait recipe add 1 nip (30mL) of your favourite liqueur prior to serving.

CHAPTER

5

DIET FOR THE PERSON WITH A KIDNEY TRANSPLANT

The healthy diet pyramid	128
Eat most	128
Eat least	130
Salt	130
Alcohol	131

Initially after your kidney transplant it may be necessary to maintain some dietary restrictions. Once the new kidney is functioning normally these restrictions will no longer be necessary. Most people are then encouraged to follow a balanced diet.

There are several reasons why it is important for you to ensure that you are consuming a well-balanced diet after your kidney transplant.

Anti-rejection medications can change the body's needs for certain nutrients, specifically increasing the requirements for protein and calcium. Anti-rejection medications can also result in changes of appetite. Those people taking prednisone usually experience an increase in appetite and may as a result have problems with weight gain. Those taking Cyclosporin A (CSA) often have reduced appetite and may have problems with weight loss.

Diet can help maintain blood pressure, blood sugar and cholesterol levels within the normal limits. Some people may experience elevations in blood pressure, blood sugar and blood lipid (cholesterol and triglyceride) levels after transplantation. A well-balanced diet that aims to be reduced in salt, sugars and fats is helpful in keeping those levels within the normal range.

Most people prior to kidney transplantation are following a

special diet. Re-introducing previously restricted foods into the diet can be difficult, particularly if they have been avoided for several years. Many people are also confused as to what constitutes a balanced diet.

The Healthy Diet pyramid shows how the various foods can be combined to make up a healthy diet which provides all the necessary nutrients.

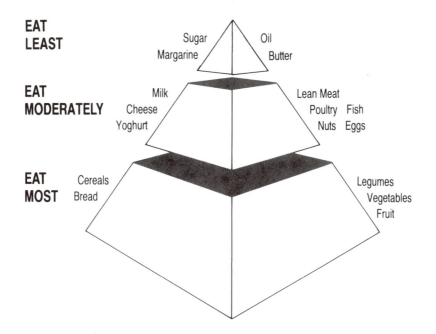

EAT MOST—BREAD, CEREALS, FRUIT, VEGETABLES

These foods are important sources of energy, complex carbohydrate, vitamins, minerals and dietary fibre. They also provide small amounts of protein.

Bread and Cereals

Three to four servings per day at least. More servings are required for active people. Wholegrain products are preferred.

Serving Size

    1 slice bread
    ½ muffin or 1 bread roll

The Person with a Kidney Transplant

¾ cup breakfast cereal
½ cup rice or pasta (cooked)
2–3 cracker biscuits

Fruit and Vegetables

Three to four servings per day. Variety provides a balance of vitamins and minerals. Include fresh as well as frozen or canned fruit and vegetables.

Serving Size

1 medium potato
½ cup vegetables
Small salad
1 piece fruit
150mL fruit juice

EAT MODERATELY—MEAT, POULTRY, SEAFOOD, EGGS, LEGUMES, NUTS, MILK, CHEESE, YOGHURT

It is important to ensure that your intake of dairy and protein foods is adequate after your kidney transplant. This is particularly important if you are taking prednisone which increases your requirement for protein and calcium. Since the waste products of protein are excreted by the kidney an adequate rather than an excessive protein intake is recommended.

Meat, Poultry, Seafood, Eggs Serving Size

2 servings per day 2 slices meat
2 small chops or small serve steak
1 medium fish fillet
¼ chicken
2 eggs.

Legumes, Nuts Serving Size

2 serves per day 1 cup cooked legumes
½ cup nuts
2 tablespoons peanut butter

Milk, Cheese, Yoghurt Serving Size

Children/adolescents—4 serves 200mL milk
Adults—3 serves 30g cheese

Pregnancy/breast feeding
Post menopause } —4 serves 200g yoghurt

EAT LEAST—FATS, BUTTER, MARGARINE, OIL, CREAM, SUGAR

Blood lipids and body weight are both elevated by excessive intakes of fat. Reducing total fat intake will help to control these. If blood cholesterol is elevated it is preferable to choose polyunsaturated or monounsaturated fats over saturated fats.

Butter, Margarine, Oil, Cream Serving Size

   1 serve per day = 1 tablespoon

Sugar

Whilst taking anti-rejection medications some people develop problems with raised blood sugar levels. This is particularly the case if they have gained excess body weight. If this is a problem reducing sugar intake will help you to decrease body weight and control blood sugar levels. See tips on reducing sugar intake.

SALT

Healthy people can obtain adequate amounts of salt in their diet from foods such as meat, milk, cereals, bread and vegetables without the use of added salt. Since the kidney is involved in regulating salt some people prior to their kidney transplant are advised to either restrict or supplement their salt intake. After transplantation salt intake needs to be reassessed.

Whilst strict restriction of salt should not be necessary after transplantation, it is a dietary guideline for all Australians to reduce their salt intake. This may be particularly relevant if blood pressure is elevated.

Salt intake may be reduced by:

1. Removing the salt shaker from the table.
2. Reducing the salt used in cooking.
3. Reducing the use of salted foods such as bacon, ham, corned beef, silverside, salted crisps and nuts.
4. Choosing reduced-salt or salt-free processed foods, e.g., reduced salt bread, margarine, butter, soups and nuts.

5. Manufacturers are required to indicate on the food label if salt is added to their product. Where possible choose products that are marked salt reduced or no added salt.

ALCOHOL

Alcoholic beverages supply few nutrients other than energy (kilojoules or calories) which comes from the alcohol and sugar they contain. Excessive alcohol intake as well as contributing to a number of diseases, accidents and social problems is also associated with lack of appetite and poor nutritional intake. Nevertheless alcohol is part of our social structure. Most health authorities recommend that two standard drinks per day such as: 2 middies of beer (2 cans low-alcohol beer); 2 nips of spirits; 2 small glasses of table wine; 2 liqueur glasses of liqueur is a safe limit for adults.

It is important to remember that alcohol is a significant source of energy (kilojoules/calories) and can contribute to weight gain. In general it is best to keep alcohol intake to a minimum.

CHAPTER

6

DIET AND FOOD PREPARATION FOR CHILDREN WITH KIDNEY DISEASE

Diet in chronic renal failure—predialysis	133
Salt	136
Potassium and fluid restriction	137
Tempting small appetites	137
Diet for the child on CAPD	137
Recipes	
Super shakes	140
High-protein cakes and biscuits	143
Breakfasts	147
Munching lunches	149
Low-protein dinners	150

DIET IN CHRONIC RENAL FAILURE—PREDIALYSIS

The aim of nutrition in children with kidney disease is to promote well-being and activity, and to improve and maintain growth.

The types, amounts and energy value (kilojoules, calories) of food eaten are an important part of their overall daily treatment. Many children have poor appetites, and are at risk of losing weight and becoming poorly nourished. The benefits of being well-nourished are many: to improve tolerance of treatment; to help fight off infection; promote growth; and to increase overall well-being. So it is important to encourage a healthy diet with plenty of high-energy foods.

Nutritional target areas for improved health and growth are:

1. Normal protein.
2. Low phosphorus.
3. High energy.
4. Low potassium.

These vary according to each child's needs.

Protein

Very low protein diets are not advised in children. This is because protein requirements are higher in childhood for growth and thus severe restriction would retard the rate of growth.

The aim is to adjust protein intake to the minimum allowance for children known as the recommended daily intake, which changes according to the age and weight of your child.

Your dietitian will calculate your child's protein requirements to meet special needs. The recipes and ideas in this book will help you to keep to the diet.

Phosphorus

The use of a low-phosphorus diet in conjunction with avoidance of high-protein diets is still at the research stage. This regimen is currently being assessed to see the effect on long-term growth rate, the prevention of renal bone disease and progression of renal failure. It is still too early to judge, but some children are showing improvement in growth and reduction in bone disease.

The main problem in restricting phosphorous in a young child's diet is cutting out milk and milk products. In many instances, children receive most of their energy from these products, and thus any phosphorus restriction would be unsuitable. Milk substitutes low in phosphorus can be recommended, but are not very tasty.

Flexibility is the key word in dietary restrictions—both protein and phosphorus are modified according to your child's eating patterns and what can be achieved practically. Your dietitian will recommend what is the best for your child.

Foods for Energy

The more high-energy foods your child eats, the more protein will be available for growth. If energy intake is too low, the body will

Children with Kidney Disease

use protein as an energy source and not for growth. It will also result in increased symptoms of kidney disease.

If the body takes in more food energy than is needed that day, the extra energy is stored in the form of body fat. This stored energy is a real bonus in times of illness or infection as it provides the body with extra fuel to help fight infection. So it is important to encourage a high energy intake as a type of insurance against the times when appetite is poor and the child is likely to lose weight.

To increase energy intake it is necessary to make sure that plenty of high-energy foods are eaten. Fat is the richest source of energy in the diet. When choosing high-energy meals and snacks, use the following guidelines.

Foods are divided into 5 food groups. These supply all the nutrients our bodies need daily. Energy-boosting ideas are given with each food group.

Energy Boosters

Breads and Cereals

Bread (try salt-free or salt-reduced varieties), breakfast cereals, oats, pasta, rice, biscuits, crumpets, pastry, scones, cakes, buns.

1. Use lots of energy-containing spreads, e.g., butter or margarine (try salt-free varieties), jam, cream, chocolate spread, honey, peanut butter (salt-free).
2. Make fried rice by frying up chopped cold meat, egg and vegetables with cooked rice.
3. Add a cream sauce or lots of butter or margarine to cooked pasta.
4. Use macaroni or rice to make high-energy milk desserts.

Fruits and Vegetables

1. Frying boosts energy, e.g., chips, stir fry vegetables, bubble and squeak, vegetable fritters.
2. Add butter or margarine to potatoes, pumpkin, peas, beans, corn on the cob, etc.
3. Use cream sauces to dress up vegetables and add energy, e.g., cauliflower, broccoli, etc.
4. Add cream, ice cream, custard to fruit. Amount will depend on protein and phosphorus restriction.
5. Glace fruits or dried fruit are very high in energy. Keep a bowl of dried fruit and nuts handy for 'nibbles'.

HEALTHY EATING ON A RENAL DIET

6. Drink cordial or fruit juice. Add a couple of teaspoons of powdered glucose to boost the energy value.

Milk Group

Milk, cheese, yoghurt, ice cream, powdered milk.

1. Do not use low-fat milk products as these are lower in energy (e.g., skim milk, cottage cheese).
2. Yoghurt is a great 'in between' snack or quick and easy dessert.
3. Use ice cream in cones for a 'between meal' treat.

Protein Foods

Serving sizes will depend on protein and phosphorus restriction.

1. Frying adds energy, e.g., home made crumbed chicken and fish, mince, hamburgers, schnitzels.
2. Fried sausages, fish fingers, and hamburgers are favourites, but commercial varieties are high in salt.
3. Baked beans.
4. Use nuts as 'in between' nibbles or in cakes and biscuits (not for children under 5, as there is a danger of choking).
5. Eggs can be given as omelettes or fried or scrambled. Try blending into milkshakes or fruit juices.

Fats and Oils

Butter, margarine, oil, cream, lard.

1. Try buying salt-free varieties of butter and margarine.
2. Use cream on desserts, fruit, scones, pancakes, etc. Sneak a tablespoon of cream into a serve of soup and custards if appetite is poor.
3. A milk substitute is often recommended for children on low protein and phosphorus diets. Use these wherever milk is indicated.

SODIUM (SALT)

Keeping a check on the salt intake of your child is important. Encourage a 'no added salt' diet, i.e., no salt during cooking or on the table. Use less of the highly salted foods, i.e. potato crisps, salted and canned meats, salted nuts, etc.

Children with Kidney Disease

We should all be following these guidelines, as one of the dietary guidelines for all Australians is to use less salt—a high salt intake is linked to high blood pressure. So, the whole family can follow a no added salt diet! Look at the guidelines on pages 4–5.

However, some children have a type of renal failure called salt-losing nephropathy which increases the amount of salt that they need. You should always check with your doctor before restricting your child's salt intake.

POTASSIUM AND FLUID RESTRICTION

Both potassium and fluid restrictions are based on the severity and type of your child's chronic renal failure. Your doctor and dietitian will recommend restrictions accordingly.

Look at the guidelines for potassium restriction on pages 56–7.

TEMPTING SMALL APPETITES

In helping your child choose high-energy meals and snacks, encourage him or her to eat more of the concentrated sources of energy, foods which pack a lot of energy and are easy to eat. Don't waste tummy space on foods that are bulky and low in energy, e.g., dry biscuits, raw vegetables—use the ideas given as much as possible.

Making food interesting and fun tempts tastebuds, e.g., cut sandwiches into animal shapes; use a 'funny' straw for milkshakes and drinks.

Only give small serves, and seconds if needed. Too much food on the plate can discourage children and put them off.

Even if the child is eating differently from the rest of the family he or she should be included at the family meal table and should not be treated differently.

Small, between-meal snacks are a way of tempting small appetites and meeting high energy needs. Snacks can easily contribute to the daily nutritional requirements if the right foods are chosen.

DIET FOR THE CHILD ON CAPD

Nutrition is an important part of your child's overall daily treatment. The nutritional targets differ from those in the predialysis phase and also from adults on CAPD.

Nutritional target areas for improved health and growth are:

HEALTHY EATING ON A RENAL DIET

1. High energy.
2. High protein.
3. No added salt.

High Energy

In comparison to adults on CAPD, obesity is rarely seen in children. In fact, appetites are often poor and food intake needs to be encouraged. Energy intake is important for general health and also for growth (just like in predialysis). Try using some of the 'energy-boosting' ideas mentioned on pages 135–6.

High Protein

Protein requirements are higher than normal as protein losses occur across the dialysis membrane. So a high-protein diet is important to make up for these losses.

One good thing about protein foods is that they are also high in energy. Try to encourage at least 3 serves of high-protein foods daily: meat, fish, lentils, dried peas, nuts, seeds, eggs. Milk and milk products are high in protein and energy and are favourites with children. Try some of the 'Supershake' recipes in this chapter. Keep a check on the amount of cheese eaten—although it is a high protein/high energy food it is also high in salt.

So, encourage protein foods throughout the day for growth and also energy.

Salt

Keeping a check on your child's salt intake is important. A high salt intake can lead to problems of fluid overload and high blood pressure. Use the guidelines on pages 4–5.

Fluid restriction will be advised by your doctor.

Potassium restriction, if necessary, will be advised by your doctor (look at the guidelines for potassium restriction on pages 56–7).

Blood tests have routinely shown that children on CAPD have high blood triglyceride and cholesterol levels. This is known as hyperlipidaemia and may be important in the development of early coronary heart disease. Studies have indicated dietary modification can reduce these levels. The guidelines are:

1. Increase your child's intake of complex carbohydrates (e.g., cereals, bread, fruit, starchy vegetables) instead of simple sugars

(e.g., cakes, biscuits) and concentrated sweets. This is often hard to achieve, especially when appetites are poor and often simple sugars are the easiest way to ensure an adequate energy intake.
2. Use polyunsaturated fats, i.e., polyunsaturated vegetable oils and polyunsaturated margarine in preference to saturated fats and butter.
3. Exercise regularly.

The recipes in this book incorporate polyunsaturated fats in place of saturated fats. Similar modifications may be made to the recipes you use at home. Discuss these guidelines with your dietitian.

Super Shakes

Banana Smoothie

SERVES 1

250mL (1 cup) milk
1 × 60g egg
100g (1 medium) banana
50g (2 tablespoons) honey
Pinch nutmeg

Blend all ingredients together until smooth. Serve chilled.

Orange Spider

SERVES 1

100g (1 medium) banana, chopped
30g (1 scoop) vanilla ice cream
125mL (½ cup) orange juice

Mix together banana and ice cream in a blender. Add orange juice and blend until frothy. Serve chilled.

Supa-Dupa Shake

SERVES 1

200mL (¾ cup) milk
10mL (2 teaspoons) flavouring
50mL (¼ cup) cream
30g (1 scoop) ice cream

Blend all ingredients together until smooth.

Variation

Try blending fresh fruit for a fruit-shake, e.g., strawberries, apple, mango, blueberries.

Egg Nog

SERVES 1

250mL (1 cup) milk
1 × 50g egg
½ teaspoon vanilla essence
30g (1 tablespoon) honey
20mL (1 tablespoon) cream

Place all ingredients into a blender and blend until smooth. Serve chilled.

High-Protein Cakes and Biscuits

Honey Loaf

SERVES 15

250mL (1 cup) milk
110g (½ cup) raw sugar
100g (⅓ cup) honey
270g (2¼ cups) wholemeal self-raising flour

Place half the milk in a saucepan with sugar and honey. Sift flour into bowl and return bran part to flour. Add warm milk and blend thoroughly. Stir in remaining milk. Pour into a greased loaf tin (14 × 21cm). Bake in a moderate oven (180°C) for 1 hour. Serve hot with margarine. Makes 15 slices.

Carrot Cake

SERVES 15

290g (2¼ cups) wholemeal self-raising flour
90g (¼ cup) raisins or dates, chopped
200g (1 cup) sugar
180g (1 cup) brown sugar, firmly packed
2 teaspoons cinnamon
80g (½ cup) unsalted peanuts, chopped
60mL (¼ cup) polyunsaturated oil
3 × 50g eggs
200g (2 cups) shredded raw carrot

In a large bowl combine all ingredients until moist, then beat with electric mixer for 3 minutes at medium speed, scraping the bowl occasionally. Pour mixture into a greased and lined 20cm square cake pan. Bake in a moderate oven (180°C) for 60 minutes or until when a skewer is inserted it comes out clean. Cool on a wire rack.

Icing

    125g (½ cup) cream cheese
    90g (½ cup) sifted icing sugar
    20g (1 tablespoon) margarine
    ½ teaspoon vanilla essence

Cream all ingredients together until light and fluffy. Spread evenly over top of cake. Makes 15 slices.

Fruit Balls

SERVES 35

    320g (2 cups) mixed fruit
    80mL (⅓ cup) apple juice
    80g (½ cup) chopped nuts (unsalted)
    40g (½ cup) coconut
    40g (½ cup) skim milk powder

Finely chop dried fruit and soak in apple juice overnight. Combine nuts, coconut, milk powder and fruit mixture and mix thoroughly. Add more milk powder if the mixture is too wet. Form into 35 balls and allow to set in refrigerator before serving.

Peanut Cookies

SERVES 30

    120g (½ cup) polyunsaturated margarine
    45g (¼ cup) brown sugar, firmly packed
    130g (1 cup) wholemeal self-raising flour
    40g (¼ cup) raw peanuts, chopped

Cream margarine and sugar in small bowl with electric mixer. Add flour and peanuts. Knead well to blend. Form into 30 balls. Place on lightly greased baking trays, allowing space for them to spread out. Press lightly with a fork. Bake in the centre of a moderate oven (180°C) for 15 minutes. Cool on trays.

Corn Flake Cookies

SERVES 30

80g (3 cups) corn flakes
40g (½ cup) coconut
90g (½ cup) brown sugar, firmly packed
120g (¾ cup) sultanas
60g (½ cup) self-raising flour, sifted
40g (4 tablespoons) full cream milk powder
125g (½ cup) polyunsaturated salt-free margarine
1 × 50g egg

Combine corn flakes, coconut, brown sugar, sultanas, sifted flour and milk powder in a basin. Mix well. Melt margarine and add to dry ingredients. Mix well. Add lightly beaten egg to mixture and mix well. Shape a teaspoonful of mixture into a ball and repeat to make 30 balls. Place onto greased oven trays, about 5cm apart to allow room for spreading, and press lightly with fork. Bake in a moderate oven (180°C) for 10 minutes or until lightly browned. Stand a few minutes on trays before lifting onto wire racks to cool.

High-Protein Cake

SERVES 24

250g (1 cup) polyunsaturated salt-free margarine
220g (1 cup) castor sugar
1 teaspoon vanilla essence
6 × 50g eggs
150g (1 cup) plain flour
150g (1 cup) self-raising flour
60g (½ cup) full-cream milk powder
180mL (¾ cup) evaporated milk
400g (2 ½ cups) sultanas

Line and grease a 23cm square cake pan and preheat oven to 180°C. Cream margarine, sugar and vanilla essence until light and fluffy. Add eggs, one at a time, beating well after each addition. Sift flour and milk powder and fold in gently, alternately with milk. Add sultanas while folding in flour. Place mixture in pan and bake 1 hour and 10 minutes or until cooked. When cooked, sides will shrink from the tin. Ice and serve sliced with margarine.

High-Protein Custard

SERVES 2

250mL (1 cup) milk
30g (2 tablespoons) custard powder
20g (1 tablespoon) sugar
1 × 50g egg
120g (½ cup) glucose polymer or glucose

Blend all ingredients together. Stir over a low heat until mixture thickens. If custard goes lumpy blend again until smooth (this must boil to rid custard of cornflour taste). Pour into serving dish.

Breakfasts

Toasted Muesli

SERVES 7

90g (1 cup) rolled oats
10g (2 tablespoons) wheatgerm
5g (1 tablespoon) bran breakfast cereal
5g (1 tablespoon) coconut
20g (2 tablespoons) chopped nuts
35g (¼ cup) sunflower seeds
40g (2 tablespoons) polyunsaturated oil
30g (1½ tablespoons) polyunsaturated salt-free margarine
40g (¼ cup) chopped mixed fruit

Combine all ingredients except dried fruit in a baking dish. Bake in a moderate oven (180°C), stirring every 5 minutes, for 30 minutes. Add dried fruit. Serve with sliced banana and milk, or add a dash of cream or yoghurt.

In winter, cook the muesli with milk for a nice change.

1 serve = ½ cup.

Pancakes

SERVES 20

150g (1¼ cups) plain flour
1 × 50g egg
375mL (1½ cups) milk
30g (1½ tablespoon) polyunsaturated salt-free margarine, melted
Oil for frying

Put the flour in a bowl, break in the egg and add a little of the milk. Beat to a smooth paste, then pour in the rest of the milk and melted margarine. Allow the mixture to rest for half an hour or so, then heat oil in a fry pan. Pour in a little of the batter and rotate pan to spead evenly. Cook for about 1 minute or until brown, turn and brown other side. Repeat with remaining mixture. When cooked, try any of the following fillings for a scrumptious breakfast.

Fabulous Fillings

CREAM SAUCE

    30g (1½ tablespoons) polyunsaturated salt-free margarine
    20g (1½ tablespoons) plain flour
    125mL (½ cup) water
    75mL (⅓ cup) cream

Melt margarine. Stir in flour over a low heat and cook for 1 minute. Mix water and cream together and gradually stir into mixture over a low heat. Continue stirring until mixture thickens.
Add any of the following:

- mushrooms (fried)
- sweetcorn
- grated cheese and spring onions

Vegetable Pancakes

Add 1 cup grated potato, carrot or zucchini to pancake mixture.

Toasty Toppings

Try one of these toasty toppings. The quantities given will top 2 slices of bread spread with 2 teaspoons polyunsaturated salt-free margarine.

Vegetables

    105g (½ cup) mashed potato
    85g (¼ cup) cooked peas
    30g (1 tablespoon) grated carrot
    ½ × 50g egg or 1 egg white or 1 egg yoke

Mix together all the topping ingredients and spread over toast. Grill until golden brown. Any combination of leftover vegetables can be used in this way.

Egg and Cheese
>   2 × 50g eggs, poached
>   40g (2 slices) cheese

Place an egg on each slice of toast and top with a slice of cheese. Grill until cheese melts.

Peanut butter and sultanas

Mashed banana, honey and chopped nuts, e.g. walnuts

Baked beans and cheese
>   110g (1 small can) baked beans
>   40g (2 slices) cheese

Spoon half of the baked beans onto each slice of toast. Cover each with a slice of cheese and grill until cheese melts.

Egg Bread

SERVES 4

>   1 × 50g egg
>   375mL (1½ cups) milk
>   30g (2 tablespoons) grated cheese
>   10g (2 tablespoons) chopped parsley
>   20g (1 tablespoon) polyunsaturated salt-free margarine
>   200g (8 slices) bread
>   Fresh tomato wedges

Whisk together the egg, milk, grated cheese and parsley. Melt the margarine in a large frypan. Dip each slice of bread into egg mixture until soaked through. Fry bread in melted margarine until crisp and golden brown. Serve with fresh tomato wedges.

Munching Lunches

Potato Fritters

SERVES 4

150g (1 cup) potato, grated
80g (1 small) onion, grated
1 × 50g egg
10g (1 tablespoon) flour
20g (1 tablespoon) polyunsaturated salt-free margarine
40g (2 tablespoons) tomato sauce (salt free)
40g (2 tablespoons) cheese

Drain the potato and onion very well, combine with egg and flour. Melt 1 tablespoon of the margarine in a small frying pan. Spoon a quarter of the potato mixture into the pan and flatten out into a round approximately ½cm thick. Cook for 3 minutes on each side. Repeat with remaining mixture. Top with a little tomato sauce and grated cheese.

Salt-Free Peanut Butter

320g (2 cups) peanuts, unsalted
30g (1½ tablespoons) polyunsaturated oil

Mix peanuts and oil in blender. Blend until paste is smooth. Add a few drops of oil if too thick. Store in a screw-top jar. Makes 1½ cups.

Low-Protein Dinners

Spring Rolls

SERVES 6

60g (¼ cup) sliced bamboo shoots
50g (¼ cup) sliced canned mushrooms
110g (1 cup) shredded cabbage
20g (¼ cup) sliced celery
60g (½ cup) beans, frozen
80mL (4 tablespoons) oil
20mL (1 tablespoon) soya sauce
12 spring roll wrappers

Fry vegetables in hot oil, add soya sauce. Allow this mixture to cool. Place approximately 1 to 2 tablespoons of mixture in the centre of each wrapper. Fold, ensuring mixture is enclosed. Deep-fry until golden brown. Makes 12.

Spring rolls can be frozen then re-heated by frying in oil or placing in hot oven for 10 to 15 minutes.

Pizza

SERVES 12

Base

60mL (¼ cup) lukewarm water
½ teaspoon sugar
1 sachet dried yeast
180g (1½ cups) plain flour

TOPPING

60g (3 tablespoons) tomato sauce
135g (1 medium) tomato, sliced
40g (½ small) onion, sliced
60g (1 small) capsicum, chopped
25g stuffed olives (optional)
100g pineapple pieces
Pinch oregano
Pinch mixed herbs

Mix warm water and sugar together, sprinkle yeast on top and let stand until foamy. Make a well in flour and pour in yeast mixture. Knead together to form a dough (may need a little extra water). Allow dough to prove for 20 minutes in a warm place. Punch down, knead and spread dough evenly into a lightly greased large pizza tray or swiss roll tin. Brush lightly with oil. Bake in a moderate (180°C) oven for 20 minutes.

Spread tomato sauce evenly over pizza base and arrange remaining topping ingredients as desired. Return to oven for further 20 minutes. Cut into 12 equal slices and serve.

Hamburgers

SERVES 6

38g (1½ slices) white bread
190g mince
75g (⅓ cup) boiled white rice
50g (½ small) onion
½ teaspoon mixed herbs
Pepper
Paprika
½ egg white, lightly beaten
10g (½ tablespoon) Worcestershire sauce

Pull bread apart into large breadcrumbs. Combine all ingredients and divide into 12 equal hamburgers. These freeze well raw (wrapped individually). Fry in oil.

Vegetable Sausages

SERVES 9

90g (1 small) onion, chopped
1 clove garlic, crushed
20g (1 tablespoon) polyunsaturated salt-free margarine
120g (1½ medium) carrots, finely chopped
100mL (5 tablespoons) water
285g (1½ cups) potato, grated
2 chicken stock cubes
Pinch oregano
15g (1½ tablespoons) bread crumbs, dried
180cm sausage skin (rinse well in cold water)
Polyunsaturated oil for frying.

Saute onions and garlic in margarine until transparent. Add carrots, water and chicken stock. Simmer until carrots nearly cooked. Cool. Add the remaining ingredients and mix well. Divide sausage skin into 6 × 30cm lengths—tie one end with thread, ¾ fill sausage skin and tie other end; tie each sausage again twice making 3 sausages. Fill a large saucepan with water and bring to the boil. Drop the sausages in and simmer for 5 minutes, remove and drain. Fry in oil, browning evenly on all sides. Serve immediately or freeze individual portions in foil. (Re-heat well in foil in oven.)

CHAPTER

7

DIET FOR PERSONS WITH KIDNEY STONES

Calcium oxalate and calcium phosphate stones	153
Uric acid stones	155
Struvite stones	156

Kidney stones (renal calculi) are a problem for many people and have been recognized as such for centuries. The causes of kidney stones are thought to be many and there are several different types of stones. Different dietary factors are associated with the different kidney stones

The single most important treatment for all types of kidney stones is to *increase fluid intake.* Drink at least 2 to 3 litres of fluid spread evenly over each day. A continuous high urine flow through the kidney is essential to dilute stone-forming substances. To achieve this, drink approximately 250mL hourly during waking hours.

The best fluid to drink is water. Milk, tea, coffee, fruit juices and mineral water may have to be avoided or limited depending on the type of stones.

Increase fluid intake if the weather is hot, you sweat heavily, you are very active or you have diarrhoea or vomiting.

CALCIUM OXALATE AND CALCIUM PHOSPHATE STONES

Stones consisting of calcium with oxalate or phosphate are the most common. They can be due to increased urinary levels of calcium (hypercalciuria) or oxalate (hyperoxaluria). Dietary factors implicated in the output of large amounts of calcium include high intakes

HEALTHY EATING ON A RENAL DIET

of calcium-rich foods, high protein intakes, high salt intakes and a high intake of spicy foods.

1. If your stones are caused by a large output of calcium in the urine you would be advised to:

- Restrict your intake of calcium-rich foods (milk, yoghurt, cheese, ice cream).
- Moderate your intake of protein (meat, fish, chicken, eggs, nuts, legumes).
- Restrict your intake of salt (added salt, cooking salt and salty foods) (see pages 4–5).
- Drink lots of fluid, especially water. (Mineral water contains some calcium and salt, the amount varying according to the brand. Limit to a maximum of 2 glasses daily.)

Your daily intake should include a maximum of:
- 300mL milk daily (skim, reduced fat or whole) or substitute.
- 50g cheese or substitute.
- 300g yoghurt (low fat or whole).

A prudent meal plan would also include:
- Bread (preferably wholegrain)—4 to 6 slices per day.
- Rice, pasta, breakfast cereal (preferably wholegrain)—1 to 2 serves per day.
- Potato—1 to 2 per day.
- Vegetables—4 serves per day.
- Fruit—3 or more serves per day.
- Meat, poultry, fish—2 small serves per day.
- Egg—2 to 3 per week.
- Legumes may be used occasionally instead of meat.
- Butter or polyunsaturated margarine up to 1 tablespoon.
- Fluids (water)—2 to 3 litres at least.

You Should Avoid

- Protein or calcium enriched milks.
- Ice cream.
- Custards and milk puddings (except if from allowance).
- Nuts and seeds.
- Chocolate.

Persons with Kidney Stones

- Edible bones in fish such as salmon and tuna.
- Salt and salty foods.

2. If your stones are caused by a large amount of oxalate in the urine you would be advised to:

- Avoid oxalate-rich foods, i.e. spinach, rhubarb, beetroot, silverbeet, beans, soy beans, kidney beans, dried figs, cashews, peanuts and pecan nuts.
- Restrict tea and coffee to 2 cups of either per day. Tea is higher than coffee in oxalate.
- Avoid Vitamin C (ascorbic acid) tablets or multi-vitamins containing Vitamin C as Vitamin C is converted to oxalate in the body.
- Drink lots of water.

Apart from these considerations you should be able to follow the same diet that is recommended for all well people to maintain their health. See the diet pyramid, page 128.

URIC ACID STONES

These stones occur much less commonly and are caused by a large output of uric acid in the urine. Dietary factors implicated in the formation of these stones include a high intake of food rich in purines and a high intake of meat, chicken, fish and cereals coupled with a low intake of fruit and vegetables.

If your stones are caused by a large output of uric acid in the urine you would be advised to:

- Avoid foods high in purines (liver, kidney, brains and the offal meats, pate and liverwurst, meat extracts and gravies, anchovies, sardines, fish roe and caviar, yeast, yeast extracts such as vegemite).
- Moderate your intake of protein-rich foods (i.e. meat, fish, chicken, eggs, milk).
- Moderate your intake of cereal foods.
- Increase your intake of fruits and vegetables.
- Drink lots of fluids, especially water.

A prudent meal plan would include:

- Bread—3 slices per day
- Rice, pasta, breakfast cereal—1 serve per day
- Potato—2 or more per day
- Vegetables—4 or more serves per day
- Fruit—4 or more serves per day
- Meat, poultry, fish—1 small to medium serve only
- Egg—2 per week
- Legumes—1 serve per day if desired
- Milk (skim, reduced fat or whole)—up to 450mL per day
- Cheese (hard or low fat)—1 serve per day
- Butter or polyunsaturated margarine—1 tablespoon
- Fluids (water, tea or coffee)—at least 2 to 3 litres

STRUVITE STONES

These stones only occur in people who have repeated urinary and kidney infections and no dietary modifications are implicated.

Whatever type of stones you have and whatever special dietary modifications you must make, please remember the following points
- Keep your weight within the healthy range.
- Avoid too much fat—limit oils, butter, margarine, cream, sausages, small goods, fatty meats, pies and pastries. Use lean meat cuts, remove the skin from chicken, skim off the fat from the surface of casseroles and soups. Grill, bake, microwave or steam without added fat.
- Avoid too much sugar—limit your use of sugar, jam, honey, confectionary, soft drinks, cakes, biscuits, chocolate. Use unsweetened fruit juices and canned fruits, unsweetened breakfast cereals.
- Limit alcohol intake—no more than 2 drinks per day is suggested.
- Drink more water—keep a jug of water in the refrigerator, serve water with meals. Ask for iced water in restaurants.

APPENDICES—NUTRIENT COMPOSITION OF RECIPES

1. Low-protein recipe analysis	158
2. Haemodialysis recipe analysis	165
3. Continuous ambulatory peritoneal dialysis recipe analysis	169
4. Children's recipe analysis	174

*indicates recipe is unsuitable for low-sodium diets
†indicates recipe is unsuitable for low-potassium diets
‡indicates recipe is unsuitable for low-phosphorus diets

1. LOW-PROTEIN RECIPE ANALYSIS (PER SERVE)

Recipe	Serves	Energy (KJ)	Energy (Kcal)	Protein (g)	Fat (g)	Carbohydrate (g)	Sodium (mg)	Potassium (mg)	Phosphorous (mg)
Soups									
Basic Vegetable Stock		29	7	1	0.1	0.4	155	22	11
Creamed Asparagus Soup	4	870	210	3	20	6	145	270[†]	72[‡]
Cream of Carrot Soup	4	690	160	1.5	10	8	46	524[†]	118[‡]
Gazpacho	4	560	130	2	10	10	154	392[†]	38
Onion Soup	4	940	220	2	20	11	26	532[†]	136[‡]
Vegetable meals									
Fried Rice	4	650	155	1.7	10	15	49	175	40
Noodle–Vegetable Medley	4	830	200	2	15	14	24	235	47
Ratatouille	2	1090	260	3.5	21	18	18	700[†]	100
Rice Riojana	8	620	150	3	6	21	1	86	61
Savoury Stuffed Tomatoes	4	640	150	3	9	17	207	395[†]	60
Stuffed Capsicum	2	1050	250	3.5	13	31	136	377	90

Low-protein Recipe Analysis

Vegetable Cakes	4	1000	240	4	14	27	41	581†	100
Vegetable Croquettes	8	820	200	3	12	20	170	322	59
Vegetable Curry	8	760	180	3	6	33	220	708†	86
Vegetable Pie	6	490	120	3.5	4	20	213	677†	119‡
Meatless Meals with Alternative Protein									
Macaroni Cheese	6	1380	330	8	24	20	208	204	160‡
Parsley Scrambled Eggs	6	700	170	7	13.5	4	111	98	124‡
Potato and Carrot Pancakes	4	900	210	7.5	6	34	159	758†	192‡
Spanish Omelette	4	860	200	8	18	5	140	211	140‡
Main Meals									
Beef Curry	4	830	200	8	14	12	104	306	81
Bolognese Sauce	6	560	130	5	10	6	230	228	55
Braised Steak	4	740	180	7	14	5	29	215	93
Cabbage Rolls	4	620	150	8	7	15	138	296	96
Chicken à la king	6	1230	290	7	27	7	178	260	112‡
Chicken Slice	8	480	110	8	3	13	64	224	113‡
Curried Chicken	6	380	90	7.5	5	3	77	223	86
Lamb Shish Kebabs	4	700	170	8	2	3	35	643†	130‡

HEALTHY EATING ON A RENAL DIET

LOW-PROTEIN RECIPE ANALYSIS (PER SERVE)—continued

Recipe	Serves	Energy (KJ)	Energy (Kcal)	Protein (g)	Fat (g)	Carbohy-drate (g)	Sodium (mg)	Potassium (mg)	Phosphorous (mg)
Main Meals									
Meat Loaf	4	650	150	7.5	13	2	82	163	74
Salmon Balls	8	1466	350	7	31	13	29	380	98
Savoury Meat Balls	4	1000	240	9	19	9	20	417†	102‡
Scallop Kebabs	4	1048	476	16	16	9	168	655†	251‡
Spaghetti Bolognese	6	1310	310	10.5	11	43	231*	235	134‡
Tuna Macaroni	8	1008	241	6	16	19	50	253	76
Veal Marengo	4	320	80	8	4	2	37	270	106‡
Savoury Sauces and Dressings									
Brown Sauce	Per Table-spoon	100	20	neg	2	1	neg	neg	2
Brown Sauce Mushroom Variation	Per Table-spoon	70	20	neg	2	1	32	18	10
Brown Sauce Piquant Variation	Per Table-spoon	100	25	neg	2	1	neg	5	2
Brown Sauce Sherry Variation	Per Table-spoon	100	25	neg	2	1	1	22	3

Low-protein Recipe Analysis

Cream Dressing	Per Tablespoon	550	130	1	13	2	83	80	22	
Curry Sauce	Per Tablespoon	90	20	neg	2	1	1	13	3	
French Dressing	Per Tablespoon	180	43	neg	5	neg	neg	2	neg	
Onion Sauce	Per Tablespoon	75	18	neg	1	1	21	20	6	
Raisin Sauce	Per Tablespoon	100	25	neg	neg	7	3	42	6	
Seafood Variation	Per Tablespoon	270	65	1	5	5	170	88†	16	
Sweet and Sour Sauce	Per Tablespoon	110	30	neg	2	3	26	12	2	
Tomato Sauce	Per Tablespoon	60	15	0.5	1	1	1	57	70‡	
White Sauce	Per Tablespoon	280	70	neg	6	3	160	43	12	

Salads

Macaroni Salad	10	450	110	3	neg	23	18	260	70	
Macaroni Salad with Dressing	10	740	170	3.5	9	23	16	240	75	
Potato Salad with Dressing	4	810	190	3	12	21	27	557†	79	

LOW-PROTEIN RECIPE ANALYSIS (PER SERVE)—continued

Recipe	Serves	Energy (KJ)	Energy (Kcal)	Protein (g)	Fat (g)	Carbohy-drate (g)	Sodium (mg)	Potassium (mg)	Phosphorous (mg)
Salads									
Rice Salad with Dressing	4	830	200	2	10	25	87	133	40
Tabouli	10	170	40	3	9	20	6	226	94
Tomato and Fettuccini Salad	10	460	110	3	2	19	29	147	48
Tomato and Fettuccini Salad with French Dressing	10	940	220	3	15	20	29	150	50
Fruit Desserts									
Apple and Lemon Dessert	4	1050	250	0.5	13	37	2	190†	17
Apricot Sago	2	1290	310	1	8	61	14	346†	38
Baked Pineapple and Apples	4	610	145	1	neg	31	5	246†	18
Banana Fritters	2	1430	340	1	10	64	2	380†	35
Bananas in Sherry	4	1190	280	2	7	54	2	694†	51‡
Berry and Marshmallow Mousse	4	1030	245	2	15	23	36	269†	50‡

Low-protein Recipe Analysis

Blancmange	2	1000	240	neg	8	42	125	3	6
Lemon Cream	4	1373	328	1	18	44	20	75	17
Lemon Sorbet	4	1040	250	neg	neg	65	3	60	25
Lemon Sorbet Peach Variation	4	1200	290	0.5	neg	74	4	160†	16
Orange Au Grand Marnier	6	700	230	1.5	neg	53	3	260†	33
Creamy Desserts									
Creamed Rice	4	1220	290	2.5	16	35	174	104†	54‡
Creamed Rice Sultana Variation	4	1370	330	3	16	45	180	215†	66‡
Custard	4	2090	500	2.5	39	27	73	250†	75‡
Fruit Custard	2	1200	290	1	20	26	12	240†	30
Ice cream	4	1620	390	1.5	29	31	49	172†	47
Ice cream Coffee Variation	4	1670	398	2	29	34	65	190†	75‡
Ice cream Fruit Variation	4	1690	400	2	29	35	50	245†	59‡
Ice cream Passionfruit Variation	4	1750	420	2	29	36	55	250†	60‡

163

LOW-PROTEIN RECIPE ANALYSIS (PER SERVE)—continued

Recipe	Serves	Energy (KJ)	Energy (Kcal)	Protein (g)	Fat (g)	Carbohy-drate (g)	Sodium (mg)	Potassium (mg)	Phosphorous (mg)
Sweet Sauces									
Orange and Lemon Sauce	Per Table-spoon	190	45	neg	neg	12	neg	neg	1
Orange Cinnamon Sauce	Per Table-spoon	240	60	0.5	neg	14	1	174†	1
Biscuits and Cakes									
Apple Cake	12	1350	320	3	10	55	123	77	103‡
Carrot Cake	10	1115	265	2	13	38	125	190†	71‡
Corn Flake Biscuits	12	250	60	1.0	3	8	83	18	5
Custard Kisses	18	490	120	0.5	8	10	3	9	9
Honey Joys	18	740	180	1.0	7	29	131	29	31
Melting Moment Biscuits	16	920	220	0.5	17	17	13	46	17
Passionfruit Biscuits	38	385	90	1	6	10	37	22	28
Shortcrust Pastry		3350	800	1	41	100	855*	16	46
Sweet Variation		3390	810	1	41	110	950*	31	56‡

2. HAEMODIALYSIS RECIPE ANALYSIS (PER SERVE)

Recipe	Serves	Energy (KJ)	Energy (Kcal)	Protein (g)	Fat (g)	Carbohy-drate (g)	Sodium (mg)	Potassium (mg)	Phosphorous (mg)
Entrees									
Broccoli and Pea Vol-Au-Vents	8	800	200	3	20	10	70	120	50
Capsicum Relish Rolls	8	440	105	2	4	18	150	170	30
Eggplant and Ginger Rolls	8	550	130	3	7	17	170	200†	50
Mustard and Potato Spring Rolls	6	440	100	1	8	7	40	140	30
Vegetable Lasagne	10	680	160	4	7	20	30	253†	65‡
Main Meals									
Meat									
Apple and Pork Chop Roast	6	958	435	16	15	4	48	270	153‡
Beef Fillets with Tarragon Wine Sauce	8	1930	460	20	30	3	85	400†	220‡
Cannelloni	6	2506	600	14	46	33	209	349	224‡
Garlic Lamb Chops	6	1035	250	10	20	1.0	55	255	100
Hungarian Goulash	10	1570	370	20	30	4	90	450†	220‡

HEALTHY EATING ON A RENAL DIET

HAEMODIALYSIS RECIPE ANALYSIS (PER SERVE)—continued

Recipe	Serves	Energy (KJ)	Energy (Kcal)	Protein (g)	Fat (g)	Carbohydrate (g)	Sodium (mg)	Potassium (mg)	Phosphorous (mg)
Main Meals									
Meat									
Veal Birds	10	490	220	14	10	10	185	220	160‡
Veal Paprika	5	740	150	10	6	7	170	410†	150‡
Veal Scallopini	8	910	220	10	10	8	60	350	160‡
Poultry and Seafood									
Chicken Chinese Style	6	1160	260	20	20	4	195	330	195‡
Chicken Marengo	4	1310	330	20	20	5	100	530†	240‡
Fish Cakes	6	1370	330	20	20	30	240*	470†	100
Fish Rolls	4	500	120	15	5	3	115	430†	240‡
Fillets of Sole with Zucchini	4	1750	420	20	20	30	320*	500†	270‡
Lemon Sesame Chicken	7	690	160	20	8	5	50	240	330‡
Peppered Calamari	5	1530	365	18	28	neg	120	370	249‡
Turkey Fillets in Sour Cream	8	1790	430	20	34	10	170	330	240‡

Vegetables

Beans Oregano	4	240	56	1	4	5	4	182	30
Broccoli Florentine	8	220	50	2	10	10	225	170	80
Caramelized Carrots	4	110	30	neg	neg	7	20	90	10
Gingered Beetroot	4	540	135	1	3	30	10	100	10
Old-Fashioned Macaroni Salad	6	910	220	5	12	20	80	90	80
Pineapple and Capsicum Coleslaw	6	440	100	2	6	14	40	230	30
Scalloped Potatoes	10	720	170	2	12	14	115	125	40
Spicey Fried Corn	4	370	90	3	3	15	2	170	55

Desserts

Bandeux Aux Fruits	16	717	170	3	10	17	120	65	55‡
Biscotten Torte	8	1670	400	5	20	49	140	50	50
Creme Brulee	4	2850	680	6	55	44	195	305†	185‡
Honey and Apple Crepe Gateau	4	2210	525	8	27	65	105	280†	165‡
Strawberry Merangue Flan	8	1175	280	3	12	41	45	193†	35

HEALTHY EATING ON A RENAL DIET

HAEMODIALYSIS RECIPE ANALYSIS (PER SERVE)—continued

Recipe	Serves	Energy (KJ)	Energy (Kcal)	Protein (g)	Fat (g)	Carbohy-drate (g)	Sodium (mg)	Potassium (mg)	Phosphorous (mg)
Cakes and Biscuits									
Apple Shortcakes	12	875	210	3	11	24	18	70	45
Chewy Noels	12	495	115	2	4	20	50	65	50
Cream Puffs	12	1380	330	4	28	16	150	150[†]	80[‡]
Danish Crescents	10	1540	365	6	21	39	7	140[†]	50
Ginger Slice	12	680	160	2	8	22	52	20	15
Mandarin Cake	12	1430	340	4	22	32	145	110[†]	120[‡]
Spice Bread	12	1130	270	4	1	58	140	45	10

3. CONTINUOUS AMBULATORY PERITONEAL DIALYSIS RECIPE ANALYSIS (PER SERVE)

Recipe	Serves	Energy (KJ)	Energy (Kcal)	Protein (g)	Fat (g)	Carbohy-drate (g)	Sodium (mg)	Potassium (mg)	Phosphorous (mg)
Soups and Starters									
Almond Soup	5	1130	270	13	17	19	170	720†	350‡
Cheese Fondue	—	1310	310	20	22	8	430*	160	400‡
Chicken or Beef Stock	8	29	7	1.1	0.1	0.4	105	22	10.8
Combination Seafood Soup	7	1340	320	32	13	17	430*	750†	460‡
Cream of Chicken and Corn Soup	6	890	210	21	3	23	285*	620†	290‡
Fish Stock	8	29	7	1.1	0.1	0.4	105	22	10.8
Lentil Soup	4	900	210	15	1	40	77	640†	250‡
Pea Soup	6	880	210	15	3	30	250*	550†	200‡
Red Salmon Dip	8	235	56	7	2	2	151	136	98‡
Tasty Meat and Vegetable Soup	8	620	145	18	7	4	190	355†	210‡

CONTINUOUS AMBULATORY PERITONEAL DIALYSIS RECIPE ANALYSIS (PER SERVE)—continued

Recipe	Serves	Energy (KJ)	Energy (Kcal)	Protein (g)	Fat (g)	Carbohydrate (g)	Sodium (mg)	Potassium (mg)	Phosphorous (mg)
Savoury Omelettes									
Basic Omelette	1	960	225	13	20	1	240*	130	220‡
Cheese, Mushroom and Tomato Omelette	1	1700	405	24	32	4	290*	450†	470‡
Chicken, Corn and Capsicum Omelette	1	1200	285	20	21	5	310*	320	300‡
Curried Tuna and Celery Omelette	1	1370	325	27	23	0.5	300*	440†	380‡
Ham, Asparagus and Mustard Omelette	1	1510	360	0	30	2	570*	260	290‡
Salmon and Spring Onion Omelette	1	1375	325	24	23	0.5	240*	380	380‡
Stuffed Vegetables									
Chilli Cheese Filling	1	1080	255	16	18	20	290*	630†	270‡
Creamy Chicken with Dill Filling	1	700	165	20	3	18	150	640†	190‡
Curried Salmon Filling	1	730	175	15	3	23	110	633†	180‡

Nutty Ricotta Filling	1	830	195	13	7	22	260*	670+	160‡
Pizziola	1	1580	375	23	23	20	480*	780+	380‡
Tuna Ricotta Filling	1	645	155	17	0.2	18	100	550+	170‡
Savoury Melts									
Baked Bean Melt	1	1350	320	20	21	15	617*	316	278‡
Paprika Chicken Melt	1	1130	270	17	15	17	468*	185	210‡
Pizza Melt	1	1535	365	23	23	16	650*	340	370‡
Salmon and Avocado Melt	1	1350	320	20	21	15	405*	316	278‡
Tuna and Gherkin Melt	1	1230	290	20	16	18	493*	266	282‡
Savoury Jaffles									
Baked Beans and Cheese	1	1525	363	15	20	35	625*	155	200‡
Cheese and Chutney	1	1240	295	13	12	36	600*	220	100
Cheese and Raisin	1	1325	315	13	12	41	595*	325	115‡
Cheese and Walnuts	1	1690	402	16	25	33	580*	275	185‡
Cheese, Tomato and Celery	1	1430	340	13	18	305*	655*	295	170‡
Egg	1	1250	300	12	16	29	510*	195	120‡
Ham, Cheese and Pineapple	1	1530	365	20	16	40	910*	320	140‡

CONTINUOUS AMBULATORY PERITONEAL DIALYSIS RECIPE ANALYSIS (PER SERVE)—continued

Recipe	Serves	Energy (KJ)	Energy (Kcal)	Protein (g)	Fat (g)	Carbohy-drate (g)	Sodium (mg)	Potassium (mg)	Phosphorous (mg)
Savoury Jaffles									
Salmon and Cucumber	1	1310	310	18	14	445*	290*	375	190‡
Tomato and Spring Onion	1	1340	320	22	13	30	445*	335	180‡
Desserts									
Baked Rice Custard Apple Rice Variation	4	1110	265	11	5	44	135	365+	250‡
Baked Rice Custard Artificially Sweetened	4	690	165	11	4	20	130	366+	244‡
Baked Rice Custard with Sugar	4	980	230	11	4	38	130	366+	244‡
Banana Rice Variation	4	1175	280	12	5	48	133	505+	260‡
Bread and Butter Custard Artificially Sweetened	4	860	204	13	6	24	250*	330+	250‡
Bread and Butter Custard with Sugar	4	1065	250	13	6	37	250*	330+	250‡

CAPD Recipe Analysis

Chocolate Blancmange	4	330	80	5	0	20	70	200[+]	125[‡]
Fruit Fool	4	617	145	6	0	32	115	370[+]	145[‡]
Fruit Yoghurt Ice Cream	4	610	145	11	0	24	130	430[+]	245[‡]
High-Protein Custard	4	700	165	14	0	26	210	570[+]	375[‡]
Mocha Mousse	4	525	125	12	0	16	90	410[+]	180[‡]
Pumpkin Cheesecake	12	805	190	11	8	18	255[*]	230[+]	170[‡]
Stuffed Peaches	1	535	130	4	7	15	30	295[+]	95[‡]
Tropical Fruit Yoghurt Slice	8	466	106	5	6	10	110	60	65[‡]
Beverages									
Basic Milkshake	1	1567	370	30	6	47	454[*]	1207[+]	792[‡]
Cafe Au Lait	1	356	85	9	0	12	130	360[+]	235[‡]
Fruitshake	1	1852	440	32	6	65	456[*]	1699	824[‡]
Iced Coffee	1	880	209	16	0.4	26	265[*]	658[+]	428[‡]
Liqueur Coffee	1	711	170	6.6	0.2	19	98[*]	280[+]	180[‡]
Orange Egg Nog	1	1164	277	17	6	27	291[*]	6687[+]	386[‡]
Yoghurt Shake	1	740	176	8	0.7	38	44	871[+]	153[‡]

4. CHILDREN'S RECIPE ANALYSIS (PER SERVE)

Recipe	Serves	Energy (KJ)	Energy (Kcal)	Protein (g)	Fat (g)	Carbohydrate (g)	Sodium (mg)	Potassium (mg)	Phosphorous (mg)
Supa Shakes									
Banana Smoothie	1	2207	525	17	16	80	214	883[+]	393[‡]
Egg Nog	1	1750	415	15	23	37	220	508[+]	360[‡]
Orange Spider	1	910	220	4	4	45	208	640[+]	88[+]
Supa-Dupa Shake	1	1700	405	10	31	24	173	490[+]	262[‡]
Cakes and Biscuits									
Carrot Cake	15	1124	278	5	8	46	28	194[+]	74[‡]
Carrot Cake and Icing	15	1380	330	6	12	52	72	257[+]	88[‡]
Corn Flake Cookies	30	350	83	1.0	4	10	90	74	4
Fruit Balls	35	220	52	1.6	1.6	8.9	17	130[+]	40
High-Protein Cake	24	1000	240	4.5	11	32	125	210[+]	85[+]
High-Protein Custard	2	832	200	8	9	16	160	160[+]	180[‡]
Honey Loaf	15	537	128	216	1	34	11	47	32
Peanut Cookies	30	230	54	1.0	4	5	40	14	10

Breakfasts

Cream Sauce		230	50	neg	50	1	5	10	6
Egg Bread	4	1300	310	12	14	35	500*	270+	120‡
Pancakes	20	330	79	2	5	7	24	41	33
Sauce and Cheese Spring Onions		448	107	5	9	1	134	29	106‡
Sauce and Corn		249	59	1	3	8	12.9	47	18
Sauce and Mushrooms		122	29	0.6	3	1	14	100	30
Toasted Muesli	7	726	173	4	11	16	17	173	114‡
Toasty Topping—Baked Beans and Cheese	1	1968	470	22	24	46	1133*	451†	369‡
Toasty Topping—Egg and Cheese	1	820	200	14	16	1	230	100	260‡
Toasty Topping—Mashed Banana, Honey and Nuts	1	2272	543	10	20	86	336*	582+	196‡
Toasty Topping—Peanut Butter and Sultanas	1	670	160	10	9	12	150	25	220+

175

CHILDREN'S RECIPE ANALYSIS (PER SERVE)—continued

Recipe	Serves	Energy (KJ)	Energy (Kcal)	Protein (g)	Fat (g)	Carbohy-drate (g)	Sodium (mg)	Potassium (mg)	Phosphorous (mg)
Breakfasts									
Toasty Topping—Vegetables	1	260	60	4	2	8	115	175	70
Vegetable Pancakes	20	378	90	2	5	9	60	62	36
Munching Lunches									
Potato Fritters	4	550	130	5	20	16	120	190	100
Salt-Free Peanut Butter	18	478	114	4	10	2	30	96	66
Tomato Sauce		111	27	0.2	3	1	11.9	5	2.5
Low-Protein Dinners									
Hamburgers	6	600	140	8	9	6	150	150	80
Pizza	12	606	140	4	3	30	80	90	35
Spring Rolls	6	320	76	0.6	8	2	150	80	20
Vegetable Sausages	9	232	55	2	2	9	20	195	30

INDEX

A

alcohol, and transplant 131
almond soup 107
almond torte 84
apple and honey crepe gateau 87–8
apple and lemon desert 47
apple and pineapple, baked 45
apple and pork chop roast 74–5
apple cake 54
apple rice pudding 120
apple shortcakes 91
apricot sago 43
Asian cuisine
　and CAPD 99
　and haemodialysis 58–9
asparagus soup, creamed 18
avocado and salmon melt 116

B

baked bean and cheese jaffle 117
baked bean melt 115
banana fritters 45
banana rice pudding 120
banana smoothie 140
bananas in sherry 46
bandeaux aux fruits 85
beef curry 28
beef dishes
　beef curry 28
　beef fillets with tarragon wine sauce 72
　beef stock 106
　bolognase sauce 31
　braised steak 29
　cabbage rolls 30
　Hungarian goulash 76–7
　meat loaf 30–1
beef fillets with tarragon wine sauce 72
beetroot, gingered 80–1
berry and marshmallow mousse 47
beverages
　banana smoothie 140
　cafe au lait 126
　egg nog 141
　iced coffee 126
　liqueur coffee 126
　milkshakes 125
　orange egg nog 125
　orange spider 140
　supa-dupa shake 140–1
　yoghurt shake 125
biscotten torte 84
biscuits
　apple shortcakes 91
　chewy noels 90
　corn flake biscuits 52
　corn flake cookies 144
　custard kisses 51
　Danish crescents 89
　fruit balls 143
　ginger slice 91–2
　honey joys 51
　melting moments 53
　passionfruit biscuits 52
　peanut cookies 143
blancmange 44, 121
body weight
　and fluid retention 95–6
　maintaining 96–7
bolognese sauce 31
braised steak 29
bread and butter custard 120
broccoli and pea vol-au-vents 67
broccoli, Florentine 81

C

cabbage rolls 30
cakes
　apple cake 54
　carrot cake 53, 142–3
　high-protein cake 144–5

honey loaf 142
mandarin cake 90
spice bread 89
calamari, peppered 79
cannelloni 70–1
CAPD 3, 93–4
  body weight and 95–7
  diet for children on 137–9
  and eating out 95–7
  and increased protein needs 94–5
capsicum
  and pineapple coleslaw 82
  red capsicum relish rolls 66
  stuffed 22
carbohydrate 1
  energy booster for children 135
carrot and potato pancakes 26
carrot cake 53, 142–3
carrot soup, cream of 17
carrots, caramelized 80
cheese and baked bean jaffle 117
cheese and chutney jaffle 117
cheese and raisin jaffle 117
cheese and walnut jaffle 118
cheese fondue 105
cheese, ham and pineapple jaffle 117
cheese, tomato and celery jaffle 118
cheesecake, pumpkin 123
chewy noels 90
chicken à la king 34
chicken and corn cream soup 110
chicken Chinese style 69
chicken curry 34
chicken marengo 70
chicken paprika melt 115
chicken slice 32
children with kidney disease
  diet on CAPD 137–9
  diet in chronic renal failure 133–7
chocolate blancmange 121
coffee 126
coleslaw, pineapple and capsicum 82
continuous ambulatory peritoneal
    dialysis
  see CAPD
corn and chicken cream soup 110
corn flake biscuits 52
corn flake cookies 144
corn, spicy fried 82
cream puffs 92
creamed rice 48
crème brulée 86–7

curry dishes
  beef 28
  chicken 34
  curry sauce 36
  vegetable 24
custard 49
  baked rice 119–20
  bread and butter 120
  high-protein 119, 145
custard kisses 51

D

Danish crescents 89
deserts
  apple and lemon desert 47
  apple rice pudding 120
  apricot sago 43
  baked pineapple and apples 45
  baked rice custard 119
  banana fritters 44–5
  banana rice pudding 120
  bananas in sherry 46
  bandeaux aux fruits 85
  berry and marshmallow mousse 47
  biscotten torte (almond torte) 84
  blancmange 44
  bread and butter pudding 120
  chocolate blancmange 121
  creamed rice 48
  crème brulée 86–7
  custard 49
  fruit fool 121
  fruit yoghurt ice cream 122
  high-protein custard 119, 145
  honey and apple crepe gateau 87–8
  ice cream 48–9
  lemon cream 44
  lemon sorbet 43
  mocha mousse 122
  l'orange au grand marnier 46
  pumpkin cheesecake 123
  strawberry meringue flan 86
  stuffed peaches 123
  tropical fruit slice 124
dialysis 3
dressings
  creamy salad 38–9
  French 39
  seafood 39

Index

E

eating out
  on CAPD 98–104
  on haemodialysis 58–63
  and low-protein diet 14–15
egg bread 148
egg dishes
  crème brulée 86–7
  egg bread 148
  egg nog 141
  jaffle 117
  omelette 111–12
  orange egg nog 125
  parsley scrambled eggs 27
  Spanish omelette 26
  strawberry meringue flan 86
egg jaffle 117
egg nog 141
  orange 125
eggplant and ginger rolls 68
energy
  foods for children 134–6, 137, 138
  non-protein sources 11–12

F

fat 1
  blood fats 97, 138–9
  in diet 6–7, 96
fettuccini and tomato salad 41
fibre 1
fillings, savoury 113–14
fish cakes 78
fish fillets with zucchini 77
fish rolls 78–9
fluid restriction 57–8
  and CAPD 95–6
  for children 137
  tips for 64
fondue, cheese 105
French cuisine
  and CAPD 100
  and haemodialysis 60
fried rice 20–1
fritters, potato 149
fruit balls 143
fruit flan 85
fruit fool 121
fruit slice, tropical 124

G

gazpacho 19
gherkin and tuna melt 116
ginger and eggplant rolls 68
ginger slice 91–2
Greek cuisine
  and CAPD 100–101
  and haemodialysis 58
green beans oregano 81

H

haemodialysis
  dietary considerations 55–8
  and eating out 58–63
ham, cheese and pineapple jaffle 117
hamburgers 151
Healthy Diet pyramid 128–30
high-protein cake 144–5
honey loaf 142
honey and apple crepe gateau 87–8
honey joys 51
Hungarian goulash 76–7

I

ice cream 48–9
  fruit yoghurt 122
Indian cuisine
  and CAPD 101–2
  and haemodialysis 61
international cuisine
  and CAPD 102
  and haemodialysis 61–2
Italian cuisine
  and CAPD 101
  and haemodialysis 61

J

jaffles, savoury 117–18
Japanese cuisine
  and CAPD 102
  and haemodialysis 62

K

kebabs
  lamb 31
  scallop 32–3

kidney stones, diet for 153-6
kidney transplant
  and alcohol 131
  diet and 129-30
  and salt 130
kidneys, function of 2

L

lamb chops, garlic 72-3
lamb shish kebab 31
lasagne, vegetable 65
Lebanese cuisine
  and CAPD 100-1
  and haemodialysis 60
lemon and apple desert 47
lemon cream 44
lemon sesame chicken 76
lemon sorbet 43
lentil soup 107
low-protein diet 10-13, 15-16
  eating out on a 14-15

M

macaroni cheese 25
macaroni salad 41-2
  old-fashioned 83
mandarin cake 90
marshmallow and berry mousse 47
measures xii-xiii
meat and vegetable soup 109
meat loaf 30-1
meatballs, savoury 29
melting moments 53
melts, savoury 115-16
meringue flan, strawberry 86
Mexican cuisine
  and CAPD 103
  and haemodialysis 62
milkshake 125
mincemeat dishes
  bolognese sauce 31
  cabbage rolls 30
  cannelloni 70-1
  hamburgers 151
  meat loaf 30-1
  savoury meatballs 29
mocha mousse 122

muesli, toasted 146
mustard and potato spring rolls 66-7

N

noodle-vegetable medley 23

O

omelette
  basic 111
  cheese, mushroom and tomato 112
  chicken, corn and capsicum 111
  curried tuna and celery 111
  ham, asparagus and mustard 112
  salmon and spring onion 112
onion soup 18
onions
  sauce 38
  soup 18
orange and lemon sauce 50
l'orange au grand marnier 46
orange cinnamon sauce 50
orange egg nog 125
orange spider 140

P

pancakes, savoury 26, 146-7
pancakes, sweet 87-8
parsley scrambled eggs 27
passionfruit biscuits 52
pasta dishes
  bolognese sauce 31
  cannelloni 70-1
  chicken slice 32
  macaroni cheese 25
  macaroni salad 40-1, 83
  noodle-vegetable medley 23
  tomato and fettucine 41
  tuna macaroni 35
  vegetable lasagne 65
pastry
  choux 92
  shortcrust 54
pea and broccoli vol-au-vents 67
peaches, stuffed 123
peanut butter, salt-free 149
peanut cookies 143
pea soup 108

Index

phosphorous
  and children 134
  food list for 13–14
  low level diets 13
pineapple and apple, baked 45
pineapple and capsicum coleslaw 82
pineapple, cheese and ham jaffle 117
pizza 150–1
pizza melt 115
pork chop and apple roast 74–5
potato and carrot pancakes 26
potassium 3
  and children 137
  dietary control of 55–7, 63–4
  and sodium 5, 57
potatoes
  and carrot pancakes 26
  fritters 149
  and mustard spring rolls 66–7
  salad 42
  scalloped 80
poultry dishes
  chicken à la king 34
  chicken Chinese style 69
  chicken marengo 70
  chicken slice 32
  chicken stock 106
  cream of chicken and corn soup 110
  curried chicken 34
  lemon sesame chicken 76
  turkey fillets in sour cream 75
protein 1
  for children 134, 138
  increasing intake of 94–5
  modifying intake of 2–3, 57
  types of 10–11
  see also low-protein diet; specific recipes
pumpkin cheesecake 123

R

raisin and cheese jaffle 117
ratatouille 20
recipe analysis
  CAPD recipes 169–73
  children's recipes 174–6
  haemodialysis recipes 165–8
  low-protein recipes 158–64
relish rolls, red capsicum 66
rice
  baked custard 119–20
  creamed (desert) 48
  fried 20–1
  riojana 21
  salad 40
  stuffed capsicum 22
riojana rice 21

S

sago, apricot 43
salads
  macaroni 41–2, 83
  pineapple and capsicum coleslaw 82
  potato 42
  rice 40
  tabouli 41
  tomato and fettuccini 41
salmon and avocado melt 116
salmon and cucumber jaffle 118
salmon balls, deep fried 33
salmon dip, red 105
salt (sodium chloride) 4
  for children 138
  and diet 4–6
  and kidney transplant 130
  see also sodium
sauces, savoury
  brown 37
  curry 36
  mushroom 38
  onion 38
  piquant 38
  raisin 38
  sherry 38
  sweet and sour 37
  tarragon wine 72
  tomato 36
  white 25, 37
sauces, sweet 50
sausages, vegetable 152
savoury stuffed tomatoes 24
scallop kebabs 32–3
seafood dishes
  combination seafood soup 108–9
  deep-fried salmon balls 33
  fillet of fish with zucchini 77
  fish cakes 78
  fish rolls 78–9
  fish stock 106
  peppered calamari 79
  red salmon dip 105
  salmon and avocado melt 116
  salmon and cucumber jaffle 118
  scallop kebabs 32–3

tuna and gherkin melt 116
tuna and spring onion jaffle 118
tuna macaroni 35
seafood cuisine
   and CAPD 103
   and haemodialysis 62–3
seafood soup, combination 108–9
smoothie, banana 140
sodium 4
   and children 136–7
   dietary control of 4–6, 63–4
   and potassium 57
   see also potassium; salt
soups
   almond 107
   beef stock 106
   chicken stock 106
   combination seafood 108–9
   cream of carrot 17
   cream of chicken and corn 110
   creamed asparagus 18
   fish stock 106
   gazpacho 19
   lentil 107
   onion 18
   pea 108
   vegetable stock 17
Spanish omelette 26
spice bread 89
spring rolls 150
   mustard and potato 66–7
stock
   beef 106
   chicken 106
   fish 106
   vegetable 17
strawberry meringue flan 86
stuffed vegetables 113–14
sugar
   blood levels 97, 138–9
   in diet 96
supa-dupa shake 140–1

T

tabouli 41
take-away food
   and CAPD 99–100
   and haemodialysis 59
   low-protein choices 14
toasty toppings 147–8
tomato, celery and cheese jaffle 118

tomatoes
   fettuccini salad 41
   gazpacho 19
   sauce 36
   savoury, stuffed 24
toppings, for toast 147–8
tuna and gherkin melt 116
tuna and spring onion jaffle 118
tuna macaroni 35
turkey fillets in sour cream 75

V

veal dishes
   veal birds 74
   veal marengo 28
   veal paprika 73
   veal scallopini 73
vegetable and meat soup 109
vegetable cakes 21
vegetable croquettes 23
vegetable curry 24
vegetable dishes
   broccoli and pea vol-au-vent 67
   broccoli Florentine 81
   caramelized carrots 80
   eggplant and ginger rolls 68
   gingered beetroot 80–1
   green beans oregano 81
   lasagne 65
   mustard and potato spring rolls 66–7
   noodle-vegetable medley 23
   pizza 150–1
   potato and carrot pancakes 26
   ratatouille 20
   red capsicum relish rolls 66
   savoury stuffed tomatoes 24
   scalloped potatoes 80
   Spanish omelette 26
   spicy fried corn 82
   spring rolls 150
   stuffed capsicum 22
   stuffed vegetables 113–14
   vegetable cakes 21
   vegetable croquettes 23
   vegetable curry 24
   vegetable pie 22–3
   vegetable sausages 152
vegetable pie 22–3
vegetable stock 17
vegetables, and low-protein diet 15–16

Index

vegetarian cuisine
    and CAPD 103–4
    and haemodialysis 63
vol-au-vents, broccoli and pea 67

W

walnut and cheese jaffle 118
water 2
white sauce 25, 37

Y

yoghurt ice cream, fruit 122
yoghurt shakes 125

Z

zucchini with fish fillets 77